COLOUR GUIDE
Cardiology

KU-265-895

Andrew A. Grace MRCP
British Heart Foundation Research Fellow, University of Cambridge;
Honorary Senior Registrar, Papworth Hospital, Cambridge

James A. Hall MD MRCP
Consultant Cardiologist, South Tees
Cardiothoracic Unit, Middlesborough

Peter M. Schofield MD MRCP
Consultant Cardiologist, Papworth Hospital, Cambridge

Churchill Livingstone

EDINBURGH LONDON MADRID MELBOURNE NEW YORK AND TOKYO 1993

CHURCHILL LIVINGSTONE
Medical Division of Longman Group UK Limited

Distributed in the United States of America by
Churchill Livingstone Inc., 650 Avenue of the Americas,
New York, N.Y. 10011, and by associated companies,
branches and representatives throughout the world.

First published 1993

ISBN 0-443-04592-5

British Library Cataloguing in Publication Data
A catalogue record for this book is available from the British
Library.

Library of Congress Cataloging in Publication Data
A catalogue record for this book is available from the Library
of Congress.

For Churchill Livingstone
Publisher
Laurence Hunter
Project Editor
Jim Killgore
Production
Nancy Henry
Designer
Design Resources Unit
Sales Promotion Executive
Marion Pollock

The
publisher's
policy is to use
**paper manufactured
from sustainable forests**

Produced by Longman Group (F.E.) Ltd.
Printed in Hong Kong

Acknowledgements

We would like to thank all our friends and colleagues, mostly from Papworth Hospital, Cambridge, who have generously provided illustrations. In particular, these include: Dr Hugh Fleming, Dr Hugh Bethell, Dr Maurice Buchalter, Dr Nat Cary, Dr Anoop Chauhan, Intervention Ltd., Dr Antoinette Kenny, Dr Rachel Jenkins, Mr Stephen Large, Dr Paul Mullins, Dr Michael Petch, Dr Len Shapiro, Dr David Stone, Dr Edward Rowland, Mr Frank Wells, Dr Mark Farrington, Medtronic Ltd., Dr Catherine Stephens, Dr Jamie Vandenberg and Mr John Wallwork.

We would also like to thank Noel Powell, Stuart Newell, Bobby Lambert, Mary Delaney and Chris Wisbey for their help. The staff of the Medical Illustration Departments at Hinchingbrooke and Addenbrooke's hospitals have been excellent throughout.

1993

A.A.G.
J.A.H.
P.M.S.

Contents

1 / Risk factors for coronary artery disease

There are five principal risk factors for the development of atherosclerosis and coronary artery disease: male sex, increasing age, smoking, hyperlipidaemia and hypertension. The last three are reversible and amenable to modification to reduce potential coronary risk.

Smoking

Cigarette smoking accounts for a significant proportion of preventable deaths due to coronary artery disease. Stopping smoking leads to a reduction in risk and should be insisted on in every patient with or without overt coronary artery disease.

Hyperlipidaemia

Raised plasma lipids are usually due to a mix of genetic (monogenic or polygenic) and environmental factors. Familial hypercholesterolaemia (FH) has been well characterized both clinically and at the molecular level. In this condition genes encode low density lipoprotein (LDL) receptors that are reduced in number or dysfunctional leading to reduced clearance of LDL cholesterol from the plasma. This results in a raised plasma cholesterol, e.g. 8–15 mmol/l in heterozygotes (incidence approximately 1/500), which is associated with the early appearance of a corneal arcus (Fig. 1), xanthelasma, tendon xanthomata and coronary artery disease. The homozygous form (incidence approximately 1/1 000 000) leads to massively increased cholesterol, e.g. 15–30mmol/l, and dramatic planar xanthomata with deposits of lipid in the aorta producing supravalvar aortic stenosis and coronary artery disease, usually first clinically apparent in childhood (Fig. 3). Other forms of hyperlipidaemia characterized by different biochemical profiles and clinical expressions also occur, albeit less commonly (Fig. 2).

Hypertension

Hypertension is established as a strong independent risk factor for coronary artery disease. Disappointingly in mild to moderate hypertension, drug treatment studies have failed to show a reduction in the risk of myocardial infarction although the risk of stroke is reduced.

Other risks

Diabetes mellitus; raised lipoprotein; obesity; socioeconomic factors and physical inactivity. These have also been demonstrated to increase the risk of coronary artery disease but have less impact (attributable risk) than the main factors above.

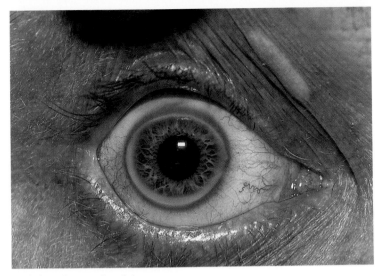

Fig. 1 Corneal arcus and xanthelasma.

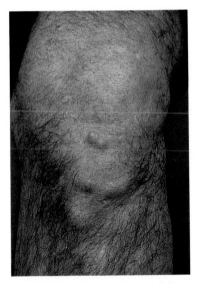

Fig. 2 Lipid deposition around the patella in type III hypercholesterolaemia.

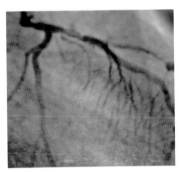

Fig. 3 Left coronary arteriogram from young patient with homozygous FH showing diffuse coronary diease.

2 / Angina pectoris

Angina pectoris is the usual symptomatic manifestation of myocardial ischaemia and results from obstructive coronary artery disease.

Terminology   ***Chronic stable angina pectoris:*** typical symptoms are predictably brought on by exercise or stress particularly in cold weather or after a heavy meal. Symptoms occur when myocardial oxygen demand outstrips supply due to a fixed atheromatous narrowing impairing flow in one or more coronary arteries.

Unstable (crescendo) angina: refers to a clinical syndrome (more akin to myocardial infarction than to chronic stable angina) where angina occurs in a rapidly progressive pattern at rest or on minimal exertion.

Variant (Prinzmetal's) angina pectoris: symptoms same in character as chronic stable angina but unpredictable in onset and unrelated to exertion. The condition is thought to arise as a result of an increase in tone in a localized segment of the coronary arterial wall.

Pathology   Coronary narrowing due to atheroma is the most common cause of angina pectoris with symptoms appearing when the lesion in a coronary artery becomes critical (usually >70% stenosis) (Figs 4 & 5). Pathological studies (Figs 6 & 7), however, emphasize that even in the presence of critical lesions the patient may be asymptomatic with the initial manifestation being sudden death.

Diagnosis   Angina is most frequently described as a central substernal dull ache with radiation to the jaw and left arm. The most important feature to establish in the history is the relationship to exercise. Rapid resolution of the symptom on stopping exertion or with sublingual nitroglycerin is often the most important diagnostic clue. However, the clinical diagnosis is never simple with 'atypical chest pain' being common and often difficult to distinguish from true angina.

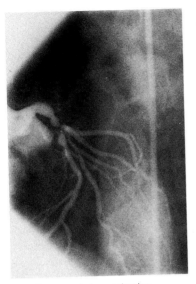

Fig. 4 Coronary arteriogram showing severe left main stem stenosis.

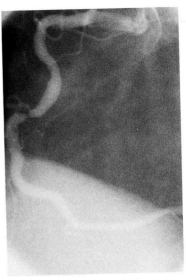

Fig. 5 Coronary stenosis in mid right coronary artery.

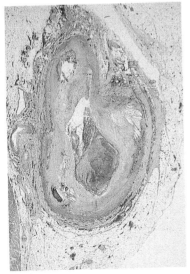

Fig. 6 Histological cross-section of an atheromatous plaque.

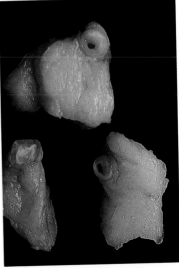

Fig. 7 Serial cross-sections through each coronary artery showing severe three vessel disease.

Basic investigations

Electrocardiography (ECG): the initial assessment of the patient with symptoms suggestive of angina pectoris should include an ECG. In the majority of patients with uncomplicated angina the ECG is normal or there are minor non-specific repolarization (ST/T) changes. The best evidence for underlying coronary artery disease in a patient with chest pain is the presence of Q waves corresponding to prior myocardial infarction which may have been clinically silent.

Chest X-ray: usually of little value in the patient with typical symptoms of angina. Patients with coronary artery disease tend to have a normal chest X-ray unless there has been a previous myocardial infarction where the cardiac silhouette may be widened due to left ventricular dilatation. Another cause for angina pectoris may be suggested by other features, e.g. aortic stenosis (valvar calcification on the lateral film) (Fig. 8).

Echocardiography: (Fig. 9) unnecessary in the majority of patients with uncomplicated angina but should be considered in specific clinical situations, e.g. elderly patients with angina and a systolic murmur (could be aortic stenosis), or with marked breathlessness or evidence of heart failure (could have left ventricular dysfunction which may be reversible).

Lipid profile: a random total cholesterol estimation is indicated in all patients with angina, especially those with clinical evidence of hypercholesterolaemia (Fig. 10). A fasting sample should be obtained if the cholesterol is raised on initial estimation to allow more precise classification of the hyperlipidaemia and selection of appropriate therapy.

Further assessment

In most patients further investigations are required to establish the presence of coronary artery disease and assess risk. These may be non-invasive, usually involving some form of stress testing which establishes the presence and extent of reversible myocardial ischaemia. Alternatively, invasive testing with coronary angiography will indicate both the presence and distribution of coronary artery narrowings.

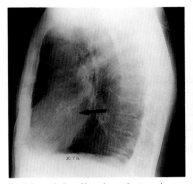

Fig. 8 Lateral chest X-ray in aortic stenosis showing valvar calcification.

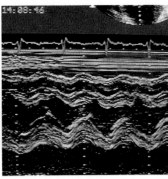

Fig. 9 M mode echocardiogram, left ventricle showing normal contraction.

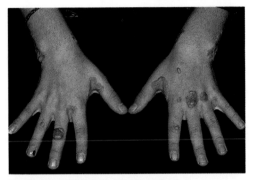

Fig. 10 Extensive planar xanthomata in familial hypercholesterolaemia.

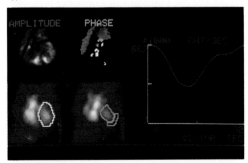

Fig. 11 Gated nuclear ventriculogram (MUGA) showing normal function (ejection fraction (EF) 53%) in a patient with angina.

Exercise electrocardiography

Principal indications
- To aid in diagnosis in patients presenting with atypical chest pain who may have coronary disease.
- To evaluate the extent of coronary artery disease (and hence prognosis) in patients with a clear diagnosis. Ideally all patients under 60 years of age and selected older patients with a history compatible with coronary artery disease should have an exercise test.
- Risk stratification following myocardial infarction.
- Provocation of arrhythmia in patients with palpitations provoked by exertion.

Contraindications
Most ambulant patients are capable of sufficient exercise to obtain a clinically useful result. Extreme caution should be observed in unstable coronary disease, severe aortic stenosis or pulmonary hypertension.

Method
Exercise level is increased on a bicycle ergometer or treadmill until a predetermined endpoint is reached or the patient develops significant symptoms (Fig. 12).

Interpretation
Symptoms and blood pressure response to exercise are also observed. For exercise to be considered adequate the patient must develop symptoms or ECG changes or reach the predetermined endpoint. Principal ECG change indicating a positive response is depression of the ST segment >0.1 mV (1 mm) (Fig. 13).

Myocardial perfusion imaging

Exercise or pharmacological stress using intravenous dipyridamole or dobutamine are used to provoke ischaemia. The test is able to distinguish ischaemic tissue from normal tissue from the distribution of isotope detected using a gamma camera (Figs 14 & 15). Reversibility also allows the investigation to differentiate ischaemic (reversible defect) from infarcted (irreversible defect) myocardium.

Indications
Patients with an abnormal resting ECG in whom changes on exercise are not interpretable (bundle branch block, ventricular hypertrophy etc.); patients unable to exercise where pharmacological stress testing is the investigation of choice, e.g. peripheral vascular disease.

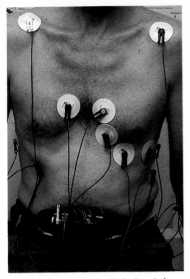

Fig. 12 Patient with leads attached ready for treadmill exercise test.

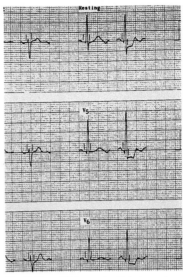

Fig. 13 Planar ST depression (right images) indicating myocardial ischaemia.

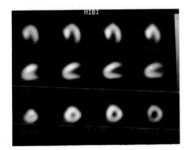

Fig. 14 Exercise perfusion study (rest image) showing normal perfusion.

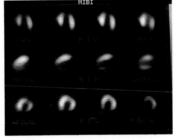

Fig. 15 Exercise perfusion study (same study showing impaired segmental inferior perfusion).

Coronary arteriography

With the development of effective non-invasive methods of assessing the presence and extent of ischaemia, cardiac catheterization is now principally indicated in patients with presumptive coronary artery disease to provide precise definition of the distribution of coronary narrowings (Fig. 16). The development of percutaneous transluminal coronary angioplasty (PTCA) has widened the requirement for the technique with approximately 600 000 procedures being carried out in the US annually.

Indications   **Establishing the diagnosis.** In patients with atypical symptoms of angina pectoris and equivocal non-invasive investigations, arteriography provides the only method of defining the diagnosis.

Determining prognosis. In patients with evidence of readily provoked ischaemia, e.g. following myocardial infarction, arteriography allows optimal management. Prognosis is principally determined by the extent of coronary disease and left ventricular function.

Planning therapy. In patients who have an inadequate response to drug therapy, arteriography allows the feasibility and advisability of revascularization with angioplasty (Fig. 17) or bypass surgery to be assessed.

Technique   The procedure is carried out under local anaesthetic. Arterial access is usually obtained via right femoral artery puncture or by cutdown onto the right brachial artery. Preshaped catheters are used to selectively intubate the origins of the left and right coronary arteries and to enter the left ventricular cavity. Dye is injected through the lumen of the catheter and video and cine images obtained (Figs 16 & 17). The procedure usually takes 15–30 minutes and is well tolerated by the majority of patients.

Complications   The incidence of major complications is approximately 0.24% with mortality about 0.06%. Most complications are produced at the site of vascular access (local complications).

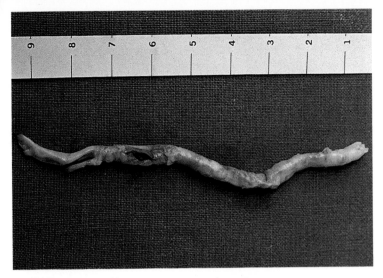

Fig. 16 Atheroma removed from coronary artery at endarterectomy.

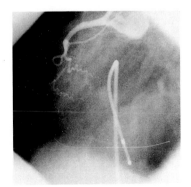

Fig. 17 Right coronary arteriogram showing occlusion of right coronary artery. Pacing wire in right ventricle. Wire passed through vessel as prelude to PTCA.

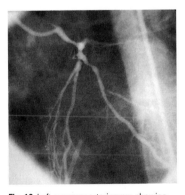

Fig. 18 Left coronary arteriogram showing disease of the left main stem and extensive involvement of the left anterior descending (LAD) and left circumflex.

Management of angina

The main objectives in the management of patients with angina are symptom relief, enhancement of prognosis and risk factor control. All patients should stop smoking, lose weight if obese and be encouraged to take regular exercise. Aspirin reduces the risk of myocardial infarction and should be given to all patients with angina in the absence of contraindications. Specific therapy must be adjusted to individual needs. Medical therapy with sublingual nitrates, beta-blockers, calcium antagonists and long acting oral nitrates is usually tried first. Patients whose symptoms are inadequately relieved should be candidates for 'revascularization' either with coronary angioplasty or bypass surgery. The two basic indications for revascularization are similarly symptom relief and improvement of prognosis.

Percutaneous transluminal coronary angioplasty (PTCA)

Procedure This procedure, like cardiac catheterization, is carried out under local anaesthetic. A fine guide wire is passed through the coronary catheter and down the coronary artery past the narrowing (Fig. 17, p. 10). A balloon catheter (Fig. 19) is passed over the guide wire and inflated (Fig. 20) squashing the atheroma, stretching the artery and relieving the obstruction (Fig. 21). The majority of angioplasties in the United Kingdom are in patients with one lesion in a single coronary artery ('single vessel disease').

Results Successful reduction of the coronary stenosis relieves angina in the majority of patients. Studies comparing angioplasty and bypass surgery as treatment of coronary artery disease are in progress.

Problems The mortality of the procedure is <1% with sudden acute reocclusion of the dilated artery being the main concern. In 20–30% of patients restenosis of the dilated vessel occurs 1–6 months following PTCA and results in a recurrence of symptoms and the need for a repeat procedure.

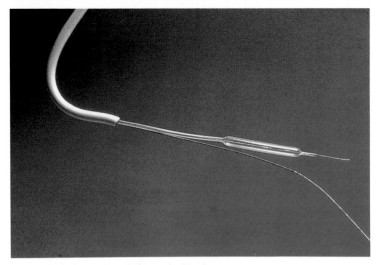

Fig. 19 Angioplasty catheter, balloon and guide wire.

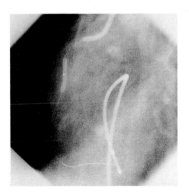

Fig. 20 PTCA showing balloon inflated at site of stenosis.

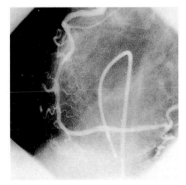

Fig. 21 Obstruction relieved, with widely patent right coronary artery.

Coronary artery bypass graft (CABG)

Indications   ***Relief of symptoms.*** CABG is a very effective method of relieving angina with >90% success rate. In the US, patients with relatively mild symptoms are operated on; however, most patients in the UK have severely disabling symptoms or are intolerant of medical therapy. Coronary bypass surgery is the most common operative procedure undertaken in the US.

Improvement of prognosis. Patients with left main stem disease, many of those with 'triple vessel disease' and some other subgroups, have an improved prognosis following CABG. Contraindications to surgery are diminishing but risk increases with impaired left ventricular function and coexistent medical problems such as cerebrovascular disease.

Procedure   The left internal mammary artery is now the 'conduit' of choice. It can, however, only be used for grafting one vessel, usually the left anterior descending artery (Fig. 22). The distal end is dissected free of the sternum and connected to the coronary artery distal to the stenosis. Most patients require multiple bypasses and lengths of saphenous vein are used, being anastomosed to the aortic root and to the distal segment of the diseased coronary artery (Figs 23 & 24).

Risks   Perioperative mortality (1–2%) is not declining as patients with more preoperative risk factors become surgical candidates. Morbidity is relatively low with the risk of significant post-bypass cerebral impairment now being established as small.

Follow-up   Coronary surgery remains palliative treatment of coronary disease. Patients require careful lifelong follow-up with particular attention being paid to secondary preventive measures. Patients should receive aspirin (if tolerated) and hyperlipidaemia should be assessed and controlled. Saphenous vein graft occlusion is inevitable and only lessened by these manoeuvres. Left internal mammary (LIMA) grafts show a strikingly higher patency rate with prolonged relief of angina and improved prognosis.

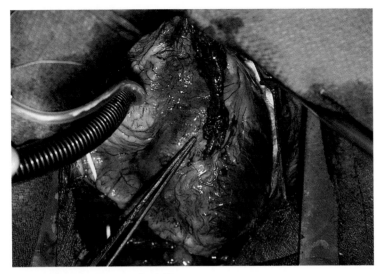

Fig. 22 Left internal mammary graft to LAD.

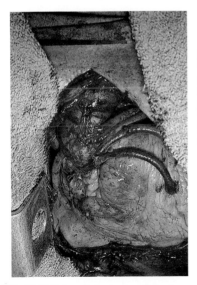

Fig. 23 Multiple saphenous vein grafts in situ.

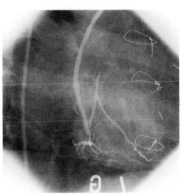

Fig. 24 Angiogram showing patent right coronary artery saphenous vein graft.

3 / Variant angina pectoris

Definition   A rare condition characterized by anginal pain occurring unpredictably at rest and often occurring at night.

Pathophysiology   Increased tone in focal segments of a coronary artery (coronary vasoconstriction) leads to reduction in flow. The mechanism of vasospasm is not entirely clear but it may be associated with vasospasm elsewhere, e.g. Raynaud's phenomenon. It may, however, complicate coronary atherosclerosis producing a mixed picture with exercise-induced angina also being combined with some unpredictability in symptoms.

Investigations   **Electrocardiography.** ECG manifestations were first described by Prinzmetal in 1959. During episodes of chest pain there is ST elevation (ST depression usually occurs with typical angina) returning to baseline as symptoms abate (Fig. 25). Episodes of ischaemia may provoke ventricular arrhythmias. ST segment change may occur in the absence of symptoms revealed particularly by ambulatory ST segment monitoring.

Coronary arteriography. This may reveal normal coronary arteries with no evidence of obstructive coronary artery disease. Coronary vasoconstriction (spasm) may be precipitated by the injection of ergonovine directly into the coronary artery with occasional dramatic consequences (Figs 26 & 27).

Management   The condition is unusual and optimal management is not established. The most common approach is to use coronary vasodilator agents such as calcium antagonists often in high doses. In the presence of coexisting obstructive disease revascularization may be necessary.

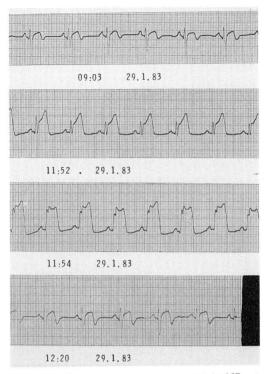

Fig. 25 ECG recorded in patient at rest showing periods of ST segment elevation associated with pain.

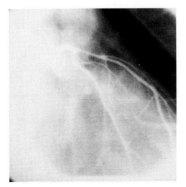

Fig. 26 Ergonovine challenge: prior to injection the LAD appears normal.

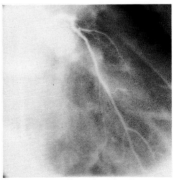

Fig. 27 Following injection of ergonovine the vessel 'disappears'.

4 / Unstable angina pectoris

Definition   Angina that is new or progresses rapidly is termed unstable angina pectoris.

Pathology   The underlying pathology is ulceration or rupture of an atheromatous plaque. Platelets adhere to the exposed collagen of the arterial wall narrowing the lumen. Vasoactive agents are released increasing smooth muscle tone with vasoconstriction further reducing flow. The process has been most explicitly illustrated in vivo by angioscopy (using fibre optic technology) although coronary arteriography will reveal an eccentric lesion with ragged edges (Fig. 28).

Investigations   **Electrocardiography.** An ECG during an episode of pain will often show ST depression with or without T wave inversion (Fig. 29). Occasionally other patterns develop such as T wave peaking or bundle branch block.

Cardiac enzymes. A patient presenting with cardiac chest pain at rest without clear-cut ECG changes of infarction may have unstable angina, be developing a 'non Q wave' myocardial infarction or be in the very early stages of a 'Q wave' myocardial infarction. These are distinguished by estimation of plasma levels of cardiac enzymes or subsequent ECG changes. Unstable angina is not associated with myocardial necrosis and there is no rise in cardiac enzymes.

Other investigations are usually of little help in planning immediate management, although an echocardiogram may show wall motion abnormalities in the ischaemic zone.

Management   Unstable angina can usually be controlled with medical therapy. Standard regimes will include oral aspirin, intravenous heparin, intravenous nitrates and oral beta-blockers and calcium antagonists. Acute intervention with angioplasty or coronary bypass may be required if symptoms prove refractory. Following resolution of the unstable phase, exercise testing is indicated to assess prognosis. Coronary arteriography is indicated if non-invasive tests or continuing symptoms suggest severe coronary artery disease (as for chronic stable angina).

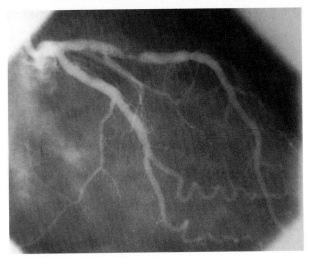

Fig. 28 Eccentric ragged LAD stenosis.

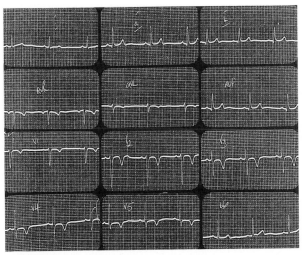

Fig. 29 ECG of non-specific changes of unstable angina pectoris (anterior T wave inversion).

5 / Myocardial infarction (MI)

Incidence Approximately 240 000 myocardial infarctions occur each year in the UK with the risk being approximately 1% per annum in middle-aged males. General practioners see on average 2–3 myocardial infarctions per annum. Early recognition is required, as 50% of all deaths occur within an hour of the onset of symptoms, although the mortality at this stage can be reduced with appropriate management.

Pathology Myocardial infarction is defined as myocardial necrosis following cessation of blood supply. The most common (>99%) cause of myocardial infarction is rupture or ulceration of an atheromatous plaque leading to localized thrombosis (Fig. 30) and coronary occlusion. Infarction is usually regional following the occlusion of a single coronary artery. Two patterns are described: either the full thickness of the myocardium is involved (Fig. 31) or necrosis is localized to the subendocardium (Fig. 32). Histological changes (Fig. 33) are not apparent for 6 hours following coronary occlusion and this has given impetus to the development of treatments which achieve early reopening of acutely occluded coronary arteries.

Diagnosis The diagnosis of myocardial infarction revolves around three criteria: history, ECG and cardiac enzyme estimation. In the early stages of evolving myocardial infarction only the first two are available.

History A typical history is available from the majority of patients, with crushing retrosternal chest pain being associated with shortness of breath, sweating, nausea and vomiting. The pain may radiate to the jaw and arms and typically builds up over several minutes to a peak. Symptoms in older patients may be atypical and not immediately referable to the heart; for example, myocardial infarction may present as an acute confusional state. Under these conditions retrospective recognition is likely and myocardial infarction is described as 'silent' (20–30% of total). It is important to carefully consider the differential diagnosis, e.g. dissecting aneurysm, gastrointestinal catastrophe, especially if the administration of thrombolytic therapy is being considered. Thrombolytic therapy should, of course, be considered in all patients.

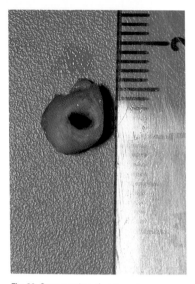

Fig. 30 Cross-section of post-mortem specimen of the LAD showing the cause of MI—intraluminal thrombus.

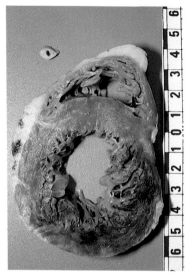

Fig. 31 Macroscopic image showing extensive transmural MI with haemorrhage and necrosis.

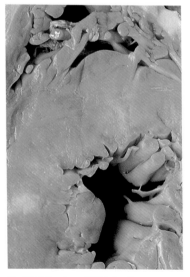

Fig. 32 Subendocardial MI showing more subtle changes confined to the subendocardium.

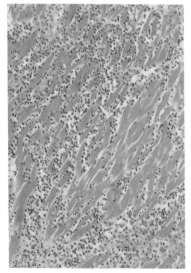

Fig. 33 Neutrophilic infiltrate in the myocardium in acute MI.

Initial investigations

Electrocardiography. It is essential to record a 12 lead ECG in patients in whom the diagnosis is considered (Figs 34, 35 & 36). ST elevation is the first change supporting the diagnosis of myocardial infarction (Q waves and T wave inversion develop later). T wave changes in isolation may be suggestive but are not diagnostic. Evolving myocardial infarction with pain is usually associated with ECG changes—chest pain and a normal ECG should suggest either alternative possible diagnoses or a request for serial ECGs.

Enzymes. Serial blood samples for enzyme estimation are usually taken and help to establish the diagnosis of myocardial infarction. The result is not usually available for 24–36 hours and therefore does not usually help early management. In patients with chest pain and regional ST elevation >1–2 mm in the limb leads or >2 mm in the precordial leads the diagnosis of myocardial infarction is virtually certain and, once the diagnosis is decided on, specific therapy should be given without delay.

Plasma lipids. Myocardial infarction is often the first manifestation of coronary artery disease, and the opportunity to obtain blood from the patient is taken to send a sample for plasma lipid estimation. The results should, however, be interpreted with caution as the stress of myocardial infarction will influence the measured values.

Further investigations

Echocardiography. In patients with uncomplicated myocardial infarction, echocardiography is not necessary. In those patients with complications manifested by cardiogenic shock, pulmonary oedema, new murmurs etc. echocardiography will provide useful diagnostic information.

Right heart catheterization. Invasive monitoring of right heart pressures and pulmonary capillary 'wedge' pressure (an index of the left heart filling pressures) by insertion of a Swan–Ganz catheter is not required in uncomplicated myocardial infarction. However, in patients with complications, e.g. shock, such information can provide useful information and guide therapy, e.g. volume expansion (in patients with predominantly right ventricular damage), vasodilatation etc.

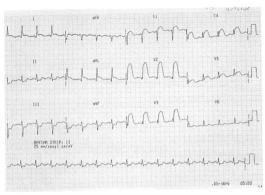

Fig. 34 ECG showing changes of hyperacute anterior MI.

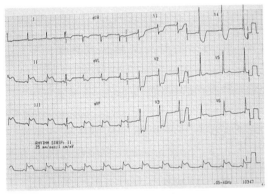

Fig. 35 Early change inferior and posterior MI.

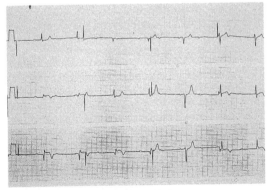

Fig. 36 Inferior MI and complete heart block.

Management of myocardial infarction

Management of acute myocardial infarction has seen dramatic changes in recent years and now, more than ever, speed in diagnosis and management are essential. If the diagnosis of myocardial infarction is suspected, all patients should be admitted to a coronary care unit, with no age limits as the elderly show most benefit.

Initial management
A defibrillator (Fig. 37) should be available as the incidence of serious ventricular arrhythmias is highest during the early phases with 25% of deaths occurring before the patient reaches hospital (Figs 38 & 39). Intravenous analgesia along with an antiemetic should be administered and oxygen given if available. Following the finding of benefit in the ISIS-2 study, aspirin is given immediately to the majority of patients.

Thrombolysis

Thrombolytic drugs can reopen an occluded coronary artery by 'lysing' occlusive thrombus, with reperfusion of the myocardium distal to the occlusion reducing infarct size. The early intravenous administration of a thrombolytic agent improves prognosis.

Indications
Provided there are no contraindications an intravenous thrombolytic agent should be given to all patients with cardiac chest pain and ST elevation or bundle branch block seen within 6 hours of the onset of symptoms. Streptokinase is given unless it has been administered in the preceding year; anti-streptokinase antibodies will be present. These antibodies increase the risk of allergy and decrease likely efficacy. In patients in whom the diagnosis is in doubt, e.g. no ECG change or non-specific findings (ST depression, T wave changes), thrombolytic therapy should be withheld and the patient observed with serial repeat ECGs. Current evidence suggests that thrombolytic therapy is probably best not given at home unless there is going to be a significant delay in transporting the patient to hospital. Other agents that may be administered once the patient has reached the hospital include intravenous heparin and an intravenous beta-blocker.

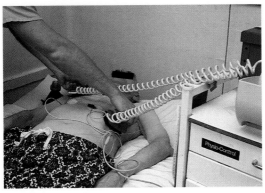

Fig. 37 Defibrillator paddles in place for cardioversion.

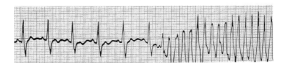

Fig. 38 Rhythm strip showing sinus rhythm degenerating to ventricular tachycardia.

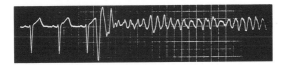

Fig. 39 R on T ectopic leading to ventricular fibrillation.

Thrombolysis (contd)

Contraindications
In general it is unsafe to give thrombolytic therapy to patients:

- with a recent history of stroke, peptic ulceration or surgery
- with a bleeding diathesis
- with proliferative diabetic retinopathy
- with severe hypertension
- during pregnancy.

Careful assessment of the history and ECG should avoid the administration to patients with aortic dissection or those with other causes of chest pain.

Complications
The major complication is bleeding. Even superficial bruising following vascular puncture may be severe, but usually more worrying is gastrointestinal blood loss or intracranial haemorrhage (Fig. 40). Other problems include those due to hypersensitivity following streptokinase, e.g. anaphylaxis, rashes (Fig. 41), proteinuria, serum sickness-like illness. As currently used, the benefits of thrombolytic therapy *far* outweigh these potential risks.

Mechanical revascularization

Angioplasty and bypass surgery have a limited role in the management of the patient following myocardial infarction. Routine use following thrombolytics is not indicated but in patients in whom thrombolysis cannot be used or those who are at high risk, e.g. cardiogenic shock, an invasive approach may offer the best hope.

Prognosis following myocardial infarction

There are three major determinants of survival following myocardial infarction:

- residual left ventricular function
- extent of underlying coronary disease
- degree of electrical instability.

Full assessment of the patient includes consideration of each of these features prior to discharge (risk stratification).

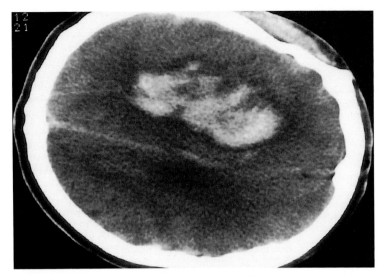

Fig. 40 Intracranial haemorrhage following the administration of tissue plasminogen activator (t-PA).

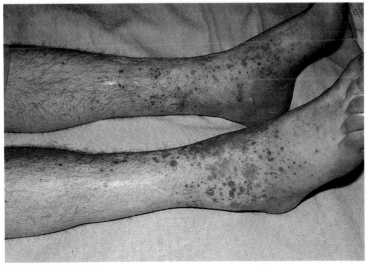

Fig. 41 Leucocytoclastic vasculitic rash following the administration of streptokinase.

Complications

Arrhythmias

Ventricular extrasystoles are very common (>90%) and in general do not require treatment. Reperfusion following thrombolysis may lead to transient sinus bradycardia or slow idioventricular rhythms and require no treatment. Tachyarrhythmias, often ventricular in origin, usually require immediate intervention particularly if there is haemodynamic deterioration. Complete heart block associated with inferior myocardial infarction is usually transient and often requires temporary pacing only (Fig. 36, p. 22). Complete heart block with anterior myocardial infarction is associated with large infarcts and a poor prognosis and will probably require permanent pacing if the patient survives.

Mechanical complications

Cardiogenic shock: associated with extensive myocardial infarction (>40% of left ventricular mass involved). The incidence remains around 7–8% and mortality >75% despite more sophisticated and aggressive therapy.

Ventricular septal defect/acute mitral regurgitation: suggested by the appearance of a new systolic murmur in a shocked patient. Diagnosis is made with echocardiography and Doppler studies with colour flow mapping (Fig. 42). Surgical repair usually offers the best chance of survival, but mortality remains around 50%.

Ventricular free wall rupture: causes 10% of in-hospital deaths following myocardial infarction. Incidence is reduced by the early administration of intravenous beta-blockers. Mortality approaches 100%. Immediate surgical repair offers the only chance of survival.

Pericarditis: acute pericarditis with chest pain and pericardial rub may occur with transmural infarction. Dressler's syndrome (fever, pericarditits, raised ESR) may appear 2–10 weeks following myocardial infarction.

Left ventricular aneurysm: develops in 8–15% patients surviving myocardial infarction.

Left ventricular thrombus: detected by echocardiography and visible on left ventricular angiography (Fig. 43) (20–40% of anterior infarcts). Embolism may cause stroke or peripheral arterial occlusion.

Deep venous thrombosis (Fig. 44).

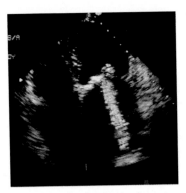

Fig. 42 Colour flow Doppler showing acute MR with jet demonstrated from the LV to the left atrium.

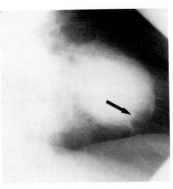

Fig. 43 Distal left ventricular thrombus shown as a filling defect on left ventricular angiography.

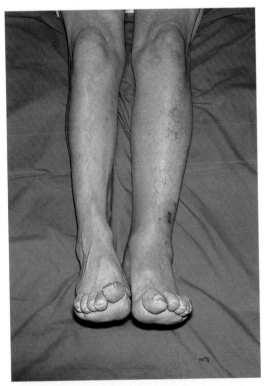

Fig. 44 Prolonged immobility following MI may lead to venous thrombosis with the risk of pulmonary embolism.

6 / Acute heart failure

Definition Acute heart failure is a sudden decline in left ventricular function usually resulting in both high filling pressures and a low cardiac output.

Aetiologhy Acute heart failure most commonly arises as a result of acute myocardial infarction, and such patients will have extensive left ventricular damage and a poor prognosis unless an acute mechanical complication of acute MI has occurred (Figs 45 & 46). In patients with chronic left ventricular disease, an arrhythmia or other circulatory stress (e.g. an infection, anaemia, minor pulmonary embolus, thyrotoxicosis) may precipitate acute heart failure. Myocarditis may present an acute picture with severe heart failure and a potentially fatal course (Fig. 47). The diagnosis of pericardial effusion with tamponade should always be considered in patients presenting with this clinical picture since it is readily treatable by pericardial drainage.

Mechanism In most patients a vicious circle of events is established where a decline in cardiac function leads to pulmonary oedema with hypoxia and to hypotension, both of which cause a fall in myocardial perfusion and further deterioration in cardiac pumping ability.

Presentation An acute onset of shortness of breath leads to patient discomfort and restlessness. Chest pain and palpitation may accompany the onset of dyspnoea and provide a useful clue to the underlying mechanism. The clinical appearance is characteristic with the patient sitting upright and using accessory muscles of respiration. The skin is pale, cool and moist. Consciousness may be obtunded.

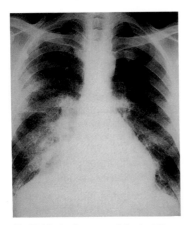 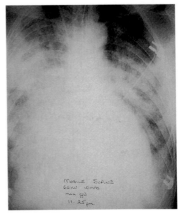

Fig. 45 Mitral valve rupture following MI showing pulmonary oedema (presentation).

Fig. 46 Same patient as in Figure 45 showing extent of deterioration 4 hours later.

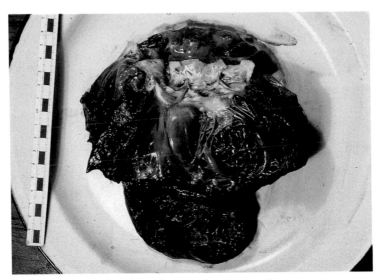

Fig. 47 Post-mortem specimen from patient presenting with myocarditis.

Examination There is tachycardia and hypotension with cool extremities due to intense vasoconstriction. Third and fourth heart sounds are usual and the jugular venous pressure may be raised. The presence of murmurs may suggest a specific cause but basal crackles lack both sensitivity and specificity in the diagnosis of pulmonary oedema. The possibility of a tension pneumothorax should always be considered. Oliguria is usual.

Investigations **Chest X-ray:** usually shows changes of pulmonary oedema with septal lines (Kerley B lines). The heart may be enlarged and evidence of a valve lesion may be present. A large globular heart shadow should suggest the possibility of a pericardial effusion.

Electrocardiography: useful in elucidating arrhythmias and establishing a diagnosis of myocardial infarction.

Echocardiography: an early echocardiogram may help to diagnose the cause of heart failure and exclude pericardial effusion (Fig. 48). Qualitative assessment of left ventricular function can be useful.

Haemodynamic monitoring: patients not responding rapidly to treatment often benefit from invasive monitoring. An arterial (radial) line to monitor systemic arterial pressure and a Swan–Ganz balloon flotation catheter to measure ventricular filling pressures are often used.

Management **General:** oxygen should be administered and assisted ventilation may be required. Intravenous diamorphine relieves distress and causes venodilatation (reducing preload).

Specific: management is determined by the initial assessment and may include intravenous frusemide and nitrates to reduce preload; correction of any arrhythmia and positive inotropes for hypotension. In patients with surgically correctable lesions the local cardiothoracic centre should be contacted for specific advice (Figs 49 & 50).

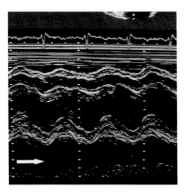

Fig. 48 M-mode echocardiogram showing large pericardial effusion (echo-Free space around heart).

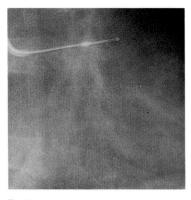

Fig. 49 Acute revascularization using atherectomy device in patient with cardiogenic shock due to acute coronary occlusion.

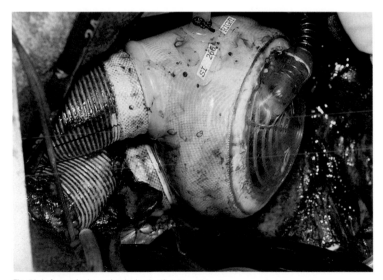

Fig. 50 Left ventricular assist device (artificial heart) in place as a prelude to cardiac transplantation.

7 / Chronic heart failure

Definition Definition remains contentious but the condition has been succinctly described as left ventricular dysfunction with symptoms. Heart failure is not a diagnosis; a specific aetiology should be established if possible. Both the incidence and the prevalence of congestive heart failure appear to be increasing. The prevalence in the UK is around 0.45% overall rising to 3% in elderly patients. 10% of people over the age of 75 are thought to have heart failure.

Aetiology The main causes are:

Coronary artery disease: causes 50–70% of cases. It is usually due to damage from prior myocardial infarction (Figs 51–54). Patients with severe coronary artery disease may have ventricular dysfunction due also to diffuse fibrosis or reversible ischaemic left ventricular dysfunction (hibernating myocardium).

Dilated cardiomyopathy: accounts for 20–30% of cases.

Hypertension: previously quoted as the most common cause of heart failure but now uncommon (<5%). The mechanism of its reduced importance as an aetiological factor is not entirely clear (p. 117).

Other causes, e.g. myocarditis, valvular heart disease, restrictive cardiomyopathy, hypertrophic cardiomyopathy, are less common (<5% in total).

Pathophysiology ***Systolic heart failure.*** The primary defect in the majority of patients is impaired cardiac contractility with a reduction in cardiac output. Secondary responses include activation of both the renin–angiotensin system and sympathetic nervous system. These compensatory mechanisms may be initially helpful but are ultimately deleterious, contributing to a progression of heart failure and increase in symptoms. Therapy is currently directed to counter the effects of these compensatory phenomena, e.g. by using ACE-inhibitors.

Diastolic heart failure. The primary defect in other patients with heart failure, e.g. with left ventricular hypertrophy, is impaired ventricular relaxation. The relative components of diastolic and systolic dysfunction are important to establish, e.g. with Doppler-echo as different approaches to therapy may be suggested.

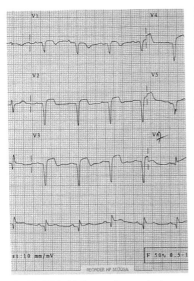

Fig. 51 ECG with Q waves in many leads indicating extensive myocardial damage.

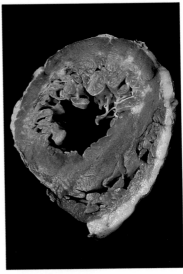

Fig. 52 Extensive old anterior myocardial infarction.

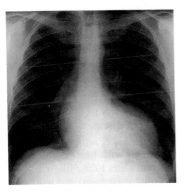

Fig. 53 Chest X-ray showing the appearances of a left ventricular aneurysm.

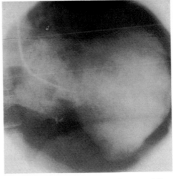

Fig. 54 Angiogram showing the same LV aneurysm as a large akinetic segment.

Assessment

Assessment of a patient with heart failure should determine the likely aetiology, determine the severity of the problem and the likely rate of progression; identify any potentially surgically remediable disease; and allow planning of therapy.

Symptoms Principal symptoms relate to fluid retention with dyspnoea, orthopnoea and ankle swelling. Symptoms of reduced cardiac output with lethargy, fatigue and mental sluggishness may also be prominent if sought.

Signs A group of signs are conventionally accepted as being indicative of the presence of ventricular failure—tachycardia, displacement of the apex beat, added third and fourth heart sounds—or represent compensatory fluid retention—raised venous pressure, peripheral oedema (Fig. 55), ascites (Fig. 56), basal crackles, palpable liver edge. None of these signs give any clue as to the underlying cause. Heart murmurs may identify valvular disease amenable to surgery, for example aortic stenosis or mitral regurgitation.

Investigations **Chest X-ray.** Any patient with breathlessness or a raised venous pressure should have a chest X-ray. The important observations in heart failure are the heart size and the presence or absence of pulmonary congestion or oedema (Fig. 57). The presence of underlying valvular heart disease or congenital heart disease may also be highlighted.

Electrocardiography. In patients with heart failure an ECG often provides important clues to the likely aetiology (previous myocardial infarction) and will identify rhythm disturbances.

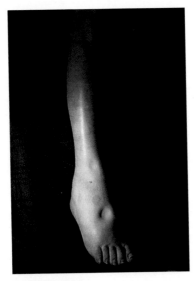

Fig. 55 Pitting oedema.

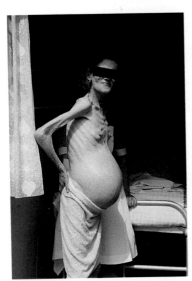

Fig. 56 Ascites associated with severe heart failure and tricuspid regurgitation.

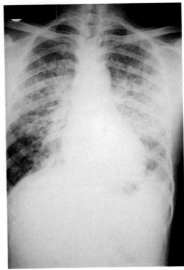

Fig. 57 Pulmonary oedema with normal heart size.

Investigations
(contd)

Echocardiography. All patients with heart failure should have a baseline echocardiogram to assess left ventricular function (Figs 58 & 59) and exclude a potentially surgically correctable cause.

Nuclear ventriculography. This remains the best way of obtaining a non-invasive quantitative estimate of left ventricular function. The result is often expressed as the ejection fraction (%) and the test also allows an estimation of the localized function of the heart. Wall motion abnormalities may be seen in coronary artery disease. The presence of left ventricular aneurysm may be indicated and suggest possible benefit from surgery (Fig. 61, p. 40).

Other techniques such as magnetic resonance imaging (MRI) may now be used to assess left ventricular function (Fig. 60) but have not yet found a role in routine clinical practice.

Prognosis

The two main predictors of outcome are left ventricular function and the presence of arrhythmia. Much of the prognostic data however relates to symptomatic status. Patients having symptoms on little exertion or at rest (New York Heart Association (NYHA) class 3–4) have an annual mortality of approximately 30–40%. This figure is comparable to many cancers. The majority of patients, however, die suddenly and are assumed to have an arrhythmia as the agonal event. The presence of arrhythmia on ambulatory electrocardiograms correlates with increased risk but suppression of these arrhythmias does not appear to improve prognosis particularly if cardiac failure is the result of myocardial infarction.

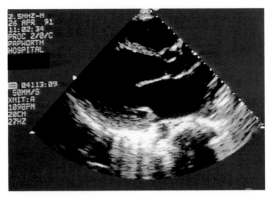

Fig. 58 2-D echocardiogram showing poor left ventricular function (systolic frame).

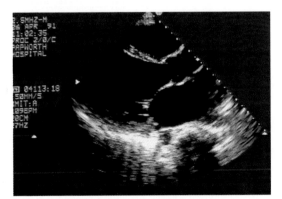

Fig. 59 2-D echocardiogram showing poor left ventricular function (diastolic frame).

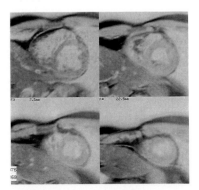

Fig. 60 Coronal section of normal left ventricular contraction demonstrated with MRI.

Management

Medical treatment

The principal aims in the treatment of chronic heart failure are to control symptoms and hence enhance the quality of life, and to improve survival. General advice should include moderate exercise that helps to prevent deconditioning and may improve outlook; cessation of smoking; and reduction of alcohol and salt intake. Drugs include:

Diuretics: the first step in most patients. They improve symptoms but have not been shown to have a beneficial effect on prognosis when used as chronic therapy, possibly due to renin–angiotensin system activation. With careful use side-effects are relatively infrequent.

Digoxin: indicated in patients in atrial fibrillation. The benefits in sinus rhythm may be trivial.

ACE inhibitors: have the advantage that they improve both symptoms and prognosis in most patients with heart failure. However, they should be used with caution, particularly in patients with coexistent peripheral vascular disease, and/or impaired renal function. Such patients may have renal artery stenosis, and precipitation of acute renal failure is possible.

Cardiac transplantation

In some patients with end stage heart failure (Fig. 61), cardiac transplantation will provide the most effective method of improving symptoms and enhancing prognosis. The resource is limited, however, by the size of the donor pool; hence patients need careful assessment and are usually not accepted if over 60 years old. Patients need lifelong treatment with immunosuppressive agents with the trend being to use low dose 'triple therapy' with cyclosporin A, azathioprine and prednisolone. Currently at Papworth Hospital the one-year survival following cardiac transplantation is 89%. Deaths in the first year are usually due to acute rejection and infection. After the first year, survival is usually good for 5–8 years, after which patients may develop coronary occlusive disease (Fig. 62).

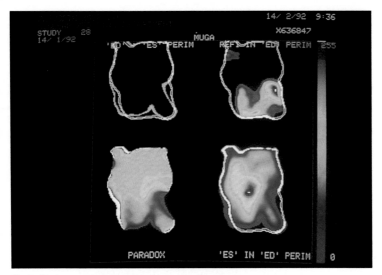

Fig. 61 Nuclear ventriculogram (MUGA) showing LV aneurysm.

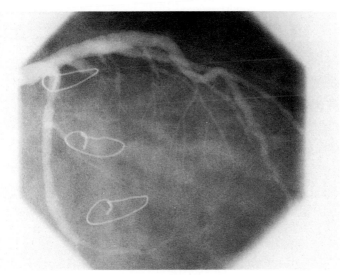

Fig. 62 Coronary occlusive disease in patient following cardiac transplantation, with tapered vessels and absent side branches.

8 / Dilated cardiomyopathy

Definition Dilated (congestive) cardiomyopathy is left ventricular dilatation with systolic dysfunction in the absence of coronary artery and valvular heart disease.

Aetiology In most patients a precise cause of dilated cardiomyopathy cannot be established. It is thought that many cases are due to previous viral infections—especially Coxsackie. Excessive alcohol consumption may lead to dilated cardiomyopathy and is important to identify as it is one of the few reversible causes. Other specific causes include nutritional deficiencies (thiamine, selenium), toxins (doxorubicidin, cobalt), specific viral infections (HIV) and infiltrations (sarcoidosis, haemochromatosis). Peripartum cardiomyopathy is a rare dilated cardiomyopathy occurring in late pregnancy or the puerperium.

Investigations **Electrocardiography:** changes non-specific and include repolarization changes, bundle branch block and atrial and ventricular arrhythmias.

Chest X-ray: cardiomegaly is usually present. Pulmonary congestion and oedema is also seen.

Echocardiography: characteristic features of a poorly functioning dilated left ventricle in the absence of regional wall motion abnormalities.

Radionuclide ventriculography: provides estimation of ejection fraction—useful prognostically (Fig. 63).

Endomyocardial biopsy: a relatively easy method of obtaining a sample of left, or more usually right (Fig. 64), ventricular myocardium for histology; only occasionally does it give a specific diagnosis (Fig. 65).

Management The treatment is that of heart failure. Anticoagulation with warfarin will protect against systemic embolism. In selected patients, beneficial effects with beta-blockers have been reported. Immunosuppressive therapy is being investigated. Transplantation may be necessary.

Prognosis Difficult to predict in individual patients, with 50% mortality in the first 2 years following diagnosis, but 25% of patients survive >10 years. Increased risk is associated with reduced ejection fraction and the presence of ventricular arrhythmias on ambulatory monitoring.

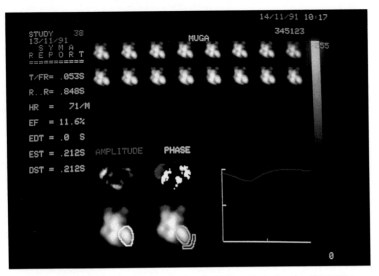

Fig. 63 Gated nuclear ventriculogram showing impaired left ventricular function (EF 11.6%) in dilated cardiomyopathy.

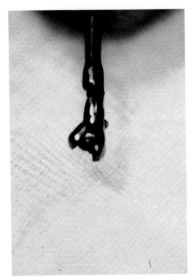

Fig. 64 Endomyocardial biopsy forceps with specimen of right ventricular myocardium.

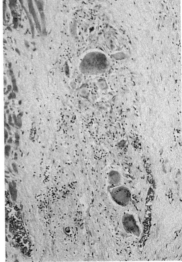

Fig. 65 Sarcoid granulomas from biopsy specimen in patient with dilated cardiomyopathy.

9 / Hypertrophic cardiomyopathy

Definition Heart muscle disease with unexplained ventricular hypertrophy, i.e. occurring in the absence of hypertension or aortic valve disease (Figs 66, 67 & 68). Symptoms arise due to obstruction to left ventricular outflow and impaired ventricular relaxation.

Aetiology 60% are familial and approximately 40% occur sporadically. Transmission is as an autosomal dominant with the gene in some families localized to short arm of chromosome 14. Penetrance in many families is high.

Clinical picture Chest pain, dyspnoea, syncope and sudden death are all features of the condition. Often patients are asymptomatic and detected on routine examination, e.g. ECG at insurance medical.

Examination Often normal. Abnormal features can include: jerky carotid upstroke, palpable atrial thrust, atrial gallop rhythm (S4) and a harsh ejection systolic murmur.

Investigations **Electrocardiography:** often very abnormal with left ventricular hypertrophy, bundle branch block, large septal 'q' waves and extensive repolarization change.

Chest X-ray: often normal. May be cardiomegaly, occasionally pulmonary oedema.

Echocardiography: diagnostic. Asymmetric hypertrophy of the ventricular septum is often seen but other distinct patterns of hypertrophy, e.g. concentric, are described.

Anbulatory ECG: indicated in all patients to establish the presence of asymptomatic atrial and ventricular arrhythmias. Non-sustained ventricular tachycardia is best predictor of risk of sudden death (Fig. 69).

Prognosis There is a risk of sudden death (2–4% per annum in adults and higher in children) and hence identification of high and low risk patients is important.

Management Symptoms may improve with calcium antagonists or beta-blockers. Diuretics and vasodilators may have an adverse symptomatic effect and digoxin is in general contraindicated. Amiodarone for patients with non-sustained ventricular tachycardia may improve prognosis. Surgery (myomectomy and/or mitral valve replacement) is occasionally required for severe outflow obstruction or mitral regurgitation.

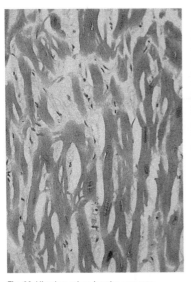

Fig. 66 Histology showing the myocyte disarray characteristic of ventricular hypertrophy.

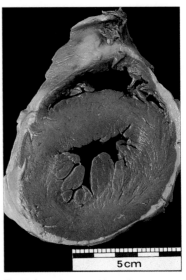

Fig. 67 Severe hypertrophic cardiomyopathy.

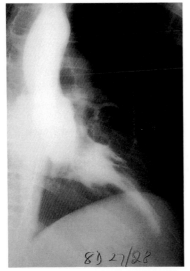

Fig. 68 Left ventricular angiogram showing characteristic appearances of hypertrophic cardiomyopathy with papillary mucle thickening.

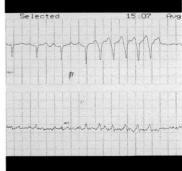

Fig. 69 Non-sustained ventricular tachycardia on ambulatory ECG recording.

Restrictive cardiomyopathy

This is a rare condition characterized by a thickened and stiff left ventricle with impaired diastolic filling. Systolic function is usually well preserved.

Aetiology No specific cause is established in most patients, but may be due to endomyocardial fibrosis or infiltration with amyloid or sarcoid, or by haemochromatosis.

Clinical picture Patients present with heart failure symptoms and a chest X-ray showing normal heart size but pulmonary congestion or oedema (Fig. 70). The appearance may be confused with lung disease, such as fibrosing alveolitis.

Investigation The diagnosis is often first suggested by echocardiography but the differentiation from constrictive pericarditis which has a similar clinical presentation is difficult and important. Distinguishing the two may require endomyocardial biopsy (Figs 71 & 72) and CT or MRI scanning.

Management Medical therapy is difficult and ultimately cardiac transplantation may be needed.

Myocarditis

Aetiology Acute inflammatory disease of the myocardium (Fig. 73) is usually due to infection with viruses (Coxsackie, echo) but occasionally due to other causes such as drug hypersensitivity or allergy (toxic myocarditis).

Clinical picture Clinical manifestations are variable with heart failure, chest pain and arrhythmias. Occasionally there is an acute presentation with rapidly progressive heart failure or shock.

Management Treatment is largely symptomatic with diuretics and ACE-inhibitors and, if necessary, inotropic and mechanical support. Spontaneous resolution may occur. Cardiac transplantation improves the outlook in selected severe cases although the use of this rare resource in sick, ventilated patients receiving inotropic support is controversial. There is no conclusive evidence of a response from immunosuppression.

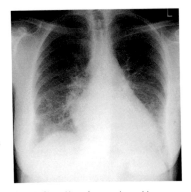

Fig. 70 Chest X-ray from patient with restrictive cardiomyopathy.

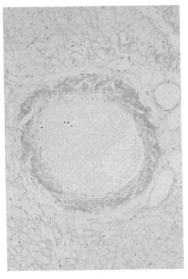

Fig. 71 Endomyocardial biopsy specimen showing amyloid (congo red).

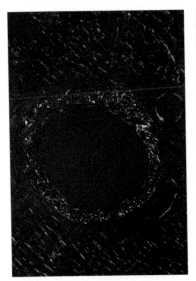

Fig. 72 Endomyocardial biopsy specimen showing amyloid (congo red polarized).

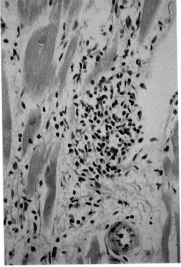

Fig. 73 Lymphocytic infiltrate of acute myocarditis.

11 / **Aortic stenosis**

Aetiology   **Congenital.** 1–2% of the population have a bicuspid aortic valve which is usually asymptomatic and associated with an ejection click and ejection systolic murmur. The valve may degenerate with calcification in adult life leading to aortic stenosis and/or regurgitation. Congenital aortic stenosis may be valvar, subvalvar or supravalvar. Supravalvar aortic stenosis may be associated with a typical 'elfin' facies (Fig. 74), mental retardation and hypercalcaemia (William's syndrome).

Degenerative. Calcific (degenerative) aortic stenosis is the most common symptomatic valve lesion seen in adult practice (Fig. 75). Approximately 50% arise secondary to a bicuspid aortic valve with the remainder occurring in normal tricuspid valves. The earliest changes, with a systolic murmur but no discernible gradient, are often referred to as aortic sclerosis.

Rheumatic. Isolated rheumatic aortic valve disease is now relatively rare and is usually 'mixed' (95%) with stenotic and regurgitant components. Coexistent mitral valve disease is usual.

Symptoms   The three classic symptoms of aortic stenosis are angina, dyspnoea and syncope. Their non-specific nature often leads to a delay in the diagnosis particularly in elderly patients in whom a high level of suspicion should be maintained. Angina may occur with normal coronary arteries as a result of an imbalance between the demand of the increased ventricular mass and the ability of the heart to supply blood but in older patients coronary artery disease is frequently present.

Signs   The most important signs are a slowly rising carotid arterial pulse, a sustained apical impulse and a systolic murmur radiating to the neck but often loudest at the apex (Gallavardin phenomenon). Clinical signs can often give an approximate indication of the severity of the disease but are frequently unreliable. Clinical assessment must therefore be confirmed using other tests (Figs 76 & 77). Hypertension in older patients with aortic stenosis is not uncommon and the pulse pressure may be wide in view of the rigid peripheral circulation. Systolic pressures of greater than 200 mmHg are, however, unusual in patients with critical aortic stenosis.

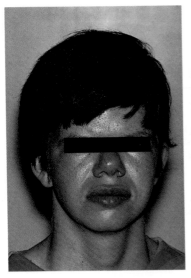

Fig. 74 Facies of supravalvar aortic stenosis.

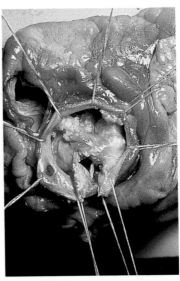

Fig. 75 Pathology of calcific aortic stenosis.

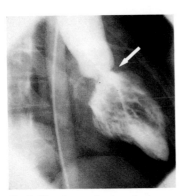

Fig. 76 LV angiogram showing subvalvar aortic stenosis.

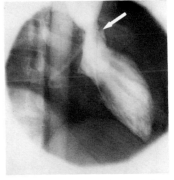

Fig. 77 LV angiogram showing supravalvar aortic stenosis.

Investigations   **Electrocardiography:** 85% of patients with significant aortic stenosis have voltage criteria of left ventricular hypertrophy (maximum S wave V_{1-3} + maximum R wave V_{4-6} >35 mm with standard ECG calibration) (Fig. 78). ST depression and T wave inversion may later develop over the lateral chest leads (V_4–V_6) referred to as a 'strain' pattern. Old anterior myocardial infarction may inappropriately be diagnosed in the light of poor anterior R wave progression.

Chest X-ray: the heart size is typically normal although a 'bulky' appearance may be suggested. The ascending aorta may be dilated proximally (post-stenotic dilatation) and is visible as a bulge at the right mediastinal border. Valve calcification is best appreciated on the lateral chest film (Fig. 8, p. 6) and its absence in a patient over 35 years of age has been said to exclude significant aortic stenosis.

Echocardiography: diagnostic investigation. It demonstrates the anatomy of the valve, indicating the extent of disruption of normal architecture (Fig. 79). Doppler study allows the measurement of the gradient across the valve (Fig. 80). Left ventricular hypertrophy is demonstrated and ventricular function may also be assessed. Some patients at low risk of coronary artery disease (young, non-smokers) may proceed to valve replacement without cardiac catheterization.

Cardiac catheterization: indicated in patients at risk of coronary artery disease in whom coronary surgery at the time of valve replacement may be needed (Fig. 81).

Natural history   Aortic stenosis typically progresses slowly and remains asymptomatic for many years. Asymptomatic individuals with mild to moderate stenosis require regular follow-up. In these individuals the risk of valve replacement outweighs any potential benefit likely from operation. Valve replacement is indicated in patients who develop symptoms and should not be delayed until irreversible ventricular damage has occurred. Aortic valvotomy (open surgery or transvenous balloon valvotomy) may be possible in young patients with congenital disease. Aortic balloon valvuloplasty is occasionally used in elderly and infirm patients in whom it may temporarily relieve symptoms although restenosis is common (>80%).

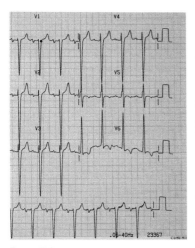

Fig. 78 ECG showing LV hypertrophy from patient with aortic stenosis.

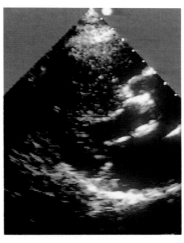

Fig. 79 2-D echocardiogram: thickened aortic valve and LV hypertrophy.

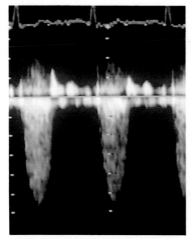

Fig. 80 Doppler gradient (>100 mmHg) across stenotic valve.

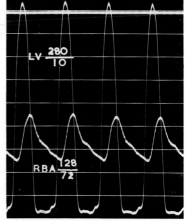

Fig. 81 Simultaneous pressure traces obtained from the brachial artery and LV showing gradient (152 mmHg).

Valve replacement

The significant advance in the management of patients with valve disease has been valve replacement.

Operation

Valve replacement is performed via a median sternotomy on cardiopulmonary bypass. The heart is arrested using cardioplegia and the operation carried out under hypothermia. The valve to be replaced is excised, and the prosthetic valve is inserted and sutured into place (Figs 83 & 84). Hospital mortality is approximately 1–4%.

Choice of valve prosthesis

Two main types of prosthetic valve are available:
- *Mechanical valves*, e.g. Starr-Edwards caged ball device, Bjork-Shiley tilting disc and St Jude bileaflet disc constitute > 60–70% valves used.
- *Tissue valves*, e.g. pig valves, cryopreserved homograft, bovine pericardium.

In general terms, mechanical valves are resilient with a low failure rate but are thrombogenic and require lifelong anticoagulation. Tissue valves have a limited lifespan and need replacement after 8–12 years; however, the incidence of embolism is lower and they may be used without anticoagulants. Tissue valves are used in patients in whom anticoagulation carries risks, e.g. a young woman who wishes to have future pregnancies.

Problems with prosthetic valves

Endocarditis: patients with prosthetic valves need to follow recommended antibiotic prophylaxis regimes.

Embolism: most dramatic manifestation is stroke but embolism to other vascular beds can also occur.

Thrombosis: valve obstruction is relatively uncommon but can follow discontinuation of anticoagulants.

Bleeding: the risk of warfarin. Lower dose regimens are now being assessed in an attempt to reduce the problem.

Prosthetic failure:
- *Mechanical*—unusual (<0.1% per annum) but catastrophic, presenting with cardiogenic shock with no audible clicks—needs immediate surgery.
- *Tissue*—failure is progressive and less dramatic. Presents with progressive stenosis or regurgitation leading to heart failure.

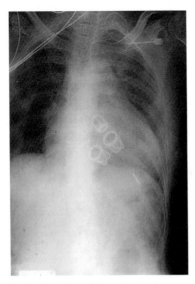

Fig. 82 Chest X-ray of three valves in situ.

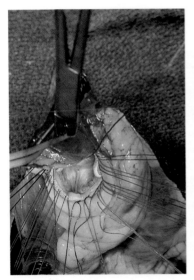

Fig. 83 Valve replacement (the operation).

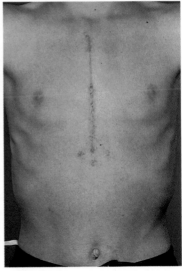

Fig. 84 The finished job—median sternotomy.

12 / **Aortic regurgitation**

Aetiology
The condition results either from a defect of valve leafets or from aortic root dilatation. Rheumatic disease and syphilis are rare causes, with infective endocarditis and idiopathic root dilatation relatively more common.

Valvar. The causes include bicuspid aortic valve (approximately 25%), infective endocarditis, myxomatous degeneration (floppy aortic valve), rheumatic heart disease (<10%) and trauma.

Root. Dilatation of the aortic root may result in the development of aortic regurgitation. Causes are legion and include annuloaortic ectasia, cystic medionecrosis (isolated or as part of Marfan syndrome; Figs 85 & 86), osteogenesis imperfecta, syphilis etc. In addition inflammatory diseases including ankylosing spondylitis, Reiter's syndrome and ulcerative colitis can be associated with dilatation of the aortic root. Acute aortic dissection may present with acute aortic regurgitation.

Symptoms
Initial symptoms in patients with chronic aortic regurgitation often relate to augmented stroke volume with complaints of a forceful heart beat and pulsations in the neck. Symptoms of heart failure ensue as the left ventricle fails. Patients with acute aortic regurgitation, e.g. infective endocarditis, may have an abrupt onset of left heart failure with vascular collapse.

Signs
With moderate to severe chronic aortic regurgitation the peripheral signs of augmented forward stroke volume are usually well marked, e.g. visible pulsations in the neck (Corrigan's sign). The pulse is collapsing in quality ('waterhammer'). The apex beat is displaced due to left ventricular dilatation and is hyperdynamic (exaggerated normal) in quality. Clinical detection relies on hearing an early diastolic murmur—heard best at the lower left sternal edge with the patient sitting up holding the breath in expiration (Fig. 87). An ejection systolic murmur is almost invariable due to the augmented stroke volume. In patients with acute aortic regurgitation the clinical signs are not usually so impressive, and the diagnosis needs careful consideration in any patient presenting with unexplained acute heart failure. The early diastolic murmur may be low pitched and difficult to hear.

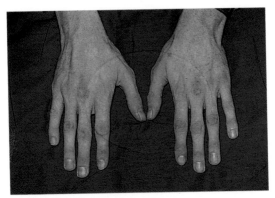

Fig. 85 Arachnodactyly (Marfan syndrome).

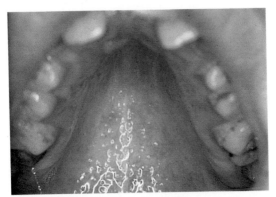

Fig. 86 High-arched palate (Marfan's syndrome).

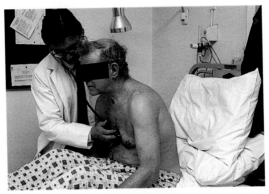

Fig. 87 Auscultation: early diastolic murmur (patient in expiration).

Investigations   **Chest X-ray:** dilatation of the aortic root is usual. Left ventricular dilatation is also present and may be marked. Cardiac enlargement is not usually a feature of acute aortic regurgitation where pulmonary oedema is more commonly seen.

Electrocardiography: left ventricular hypertrophy is usual with chronic aortic regurgitation but is not a feature of acute regurgitation.

Echocardiography: 2-D echocardiography is often useful in identifying the cause of aortic regurgitation, for example it may show aortic root dilatation, valvular vegetations or a bicuspid valve. Doppler studies are a sensitive indicator of aortic regurgitation and can provide an index of the severity of the disease (Fig. 88). Echocardiography allows serial assessment of left ventricular function. Increased left ventricular systolic dimensions are an indicator of impending irreversible dysfunction.

Aortography: classic method for defining the severity of aortic regurgitation. Dye injected into the aortic root is refluxed into the left ventricle with the volume and delay in clearance indicating the severity of regurgitation (Fig. 89).

Natural history   Chronic aortic regurgitation is characterized by an extended asymptomatic period where compensation is maintained by dilatation and hypertrophy of the left ventricle. During this phase the ejection fraction will often remain normal. Ultimately, left ventricular hypertrophy and failure supervene and correct timing of valve replacement is therefore critical.

Management   Any symptomatic patient with aortic regurgitation should undergo investigation with a view to aortic valve replacement. Patients with asymptomatic aortic regurgitation constitute a group where valve replacement may be indicated if there are signs of left ventricular dysfunction. However optimal timing of surgery in these patients is uncertain.

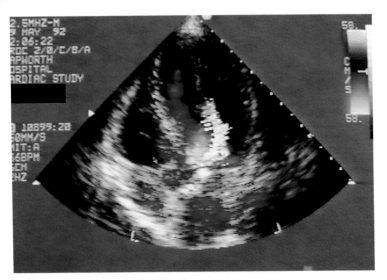

Fig. 88 Colour flow Doppler showing regurgitant jet in diastole.

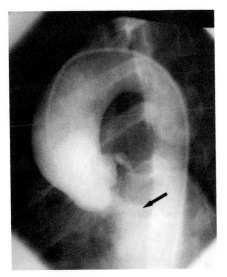

Fig. 89 Aortogram with dilatation of the aortic root and aortic regurgitation.

13 / Mitral regurgitation

Aetiology   **Coronary artery disease.** Patients with coronary artery disease develop mitral regurgitation as a consequence of left ventricular dilatation causing stretching of the valve ring, or ischaemia causing papillary muscle dysfunction.

Mitral prolapse. See page 59.

Mitral annular calcification. This is an important cause of mitral regurgitation in elderly patients occurring secondary to the deposition of calcium in the basal portions of the mitral leaflets.

Mitral regurgitation may also develop in patients with cardiomyopathy, rheumatic heart disease (usually associated with mitral stenosis), systemic lupus erythematosus (Libman–Sacks endocarditis), Marfan's syndrome, osteogenesis imperfecta and following valve destruction in endocarditis. Congenital mitral regurgitation may accompany atrial septal defects or atrioventricular septal defects.

Symptoms   Usually those of heart failure with dyspnoea and lethargy.

Signs   The characteristic finding in mitral regurgitation is a pansystolic murmur often loudest at the apex with radiation to the axilla but often heard throughout the precordium. With increasing severity there is a left ventricular gallop (S3), diastolic flow murmur and systolic thrill.

Investigations   **Chest X-ray.** Cardiomegaly is usually present with specifically left atrial and left ventricular enlargement (Figs 90 & 91). Calcification of the mitral annulus may be seen. Pulmonary congestion and oedema may be present.

Electrocardiography. Left ventricular hypertrophy is often present. In the patient remaining in sinus rhythm evidence of left atrial enlargement may be seen (P mitrale); atrial fibrillation is, however, common. The ECG may provide a clue to the aetiology, e.g. Q waves indicating prior myocardial infarction.

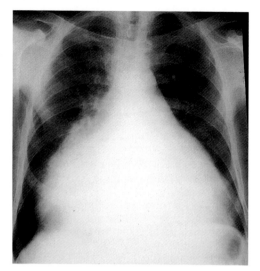

Fig. 90 'Cor bovinum'—massive cardiomegaly.

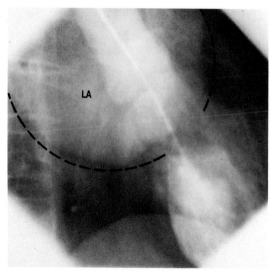

Fig. 91 Left ventricular angiogram with reflux to huge left atrium (LA).

Investigations **Echocardiography.** 2-D echocardiography demonstrates
(contd) an enlarged left atrium and hyperdynamic left ventricle
in most patients. Doppler interrogation shows a high
velocity jet in the left atrium visible in systole (Fig. 92).
Colour coded Doppler signals correlate well with
angiographic severity.

Cardiac catheterization. Left atrial pressure (pulmonary
capillary wedge pressure) is usually elevated with a
large regurgitant systolic 'v' wave (Fig. 93). Left
ventriculography demonstrates reflux from the left
ventricle to the left atrium during systole. The rate and
extent of opacification is used as an index of the severity
of regurgitation.

Natural history The natural history of mitral regurgitation is variable
and dependent on the underlying cause. Timing of
operation is controversial. Longstanding mitral
regurgitation may lead to impairment of left ventricular
function which is often not reversed by mitral valve
surgery. Therefore asymptomatic patients with severe
mitral regurgitation may be offered surgery.

Surgery Valve repair with the insertion of a prosthetic annular
ring but preservation of the integral valve structure
(Fig. 94) is becoming more common though not
applicable to all patients. Mitral valve replacement
remains the standard treatment for most patients.

Mitral valve prolapse

This is an increasingly diagnosed valve lesion. The
incidence depends on the criteria applied but ranges of
3–15% are quoted for otherwise normal women. Patients
are usually symptom free but may complain of atypical
chest pain and palpitations. A spectrum of disease exists
from mild prolapse (click only) through mild mitral
regurgitation (click + late systolic murmur) to severe
mitral regurgitation (pansystolic murmur). Severe mitral
regurgitation tends to occur in older males and may
require valve surgery. Definitive diagnosis requires
echocardiography which demonstrates mitral leaflet
prolapse in systole (Fig. 95). Patients with murmurs
require antibiotic prophylaxis against endocarditis.

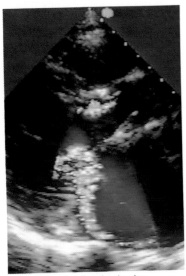

Fig. 92 Colour flow Doppler showing regurgitant jet across the mitral valve from LV to left atrium.

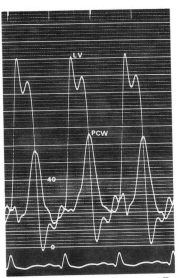

Fig. 93 Large 'v' wave in pulmonary capillary wedge pressure trace (simultaneous LV and PCWP trace).

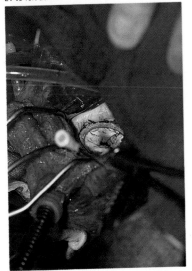

Fig. 94 Mitral valve repair with the insertion of prosthetic 'Carpentier' ring.

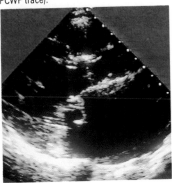

Fig. 95 2-D echocardiogram: mitral prolapse of the anterior mitral leaflet.

14 / Mitral stenosis

Aetiology   Most patients have previous rheumatic carditis though only half give such a history. Mitral stenosis results from contraction, scarring and fusion of the valve leaflets and shortening and fusion of the chordae tendineae (Fig. 96). Rare patients have congenital mitral stenosis usually in conjunction with other anomalies. Systemic lupus erythematosus, particularly when associated with circulating antiphospholipid antibodies, is an increasingly recognized, albeit rare, cause (Fig. 97).

Symptoms   Symptoms are those of pulmonary venous congestion with dyspnoea, orthopnoea and paroxysmal nocturnal dyspnoea. Pulmonary hypertension leads to right ventricular dilatation and failure with peripheral oedema and abdominal swelling. Some patients present with systemic embolism from clot arising in the left atrium. Prior to the introduction of surgery and the use of anticoagulants, >25% of deaths were due to systemic embolism.

Signs   Patients with mitral stenosis may have the mitral facies (Fig. 98) but this appearance clearly lacks specificity. Atrial fibrillation is very common and indeed usual with moderate to severe disease. The characteristic findings in mitral stenosis are on auscultation. With a mobile valve the first heart sound is loud and often palpable ('tapping' apex) with an opening snap. A low pitched diastolic rumbling murmur is heard most easily at the apex with the patient in the left lateral position. Loss of valve pliability due to calcification is usually accompanied by a loss of the opening snap and muffling of the first heart sound. Atrial myxoma may produce very similar clinical signs.

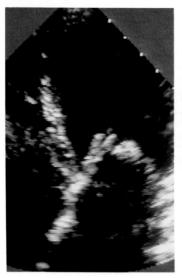

Fig. 96 Thickened dystrophic mitral valve.

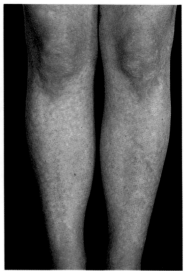

Fig. 97 Livedo reticularis in the antiphospholipid antibody syndrome.

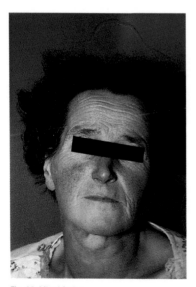

Fig. 98 Mitral facies.

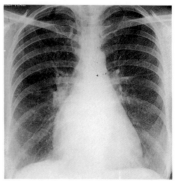

Fig. 99 Typical chest X-ray in mitral stenosis, showing straight left heart border.

Investigations

Chest X-ray. Demonstrates enlargement of the left atrium and right ventricle (Fig. 99, p. 62). Pulmonary blood flow is usually redistributed to the upper lobes and Kerley B lines develop. Chronic pulmonary interstitial oedema may lead to pulmonary haemosiderosis and ossification with small islands of bone being visible as dense nodules in the lung fields (Fig. 100).

Electrocardiography. Most patients are in atrial fibrillation. Patients in sinus rhythm show evidence of left atrial enlargement (P mitrale). Pulmonary hypertension leads to right axis deviation.

Echocardiography. 2-D echocardiography shows a deformed mitral apparatus with doming of the mitral valve. Using 2-D echo the mitral valve area may be directly planimetered. Doppler echo can assess the gradient across the valve and estimate valve area (Fig. 101).

Cardiac catheterization. A pressure gradient is present between the left atrial (pulmonary capillary wedge pressure) and left ventricular pressure during diastole (Fig. 102).

Natural history

Symptoms do not usually develop for >20 years after rheumatic carditis, after which slow development is usual.

Management

Medical. All patients with mitral stenosis and atrial fibrillation require anticoagulation to reduce the risks of systemic embolism. Digoxin is usually required for patients with atrial fibrillation to control the ventricular rates, and heart failure treatment may also be needed.

Interventional. Intervention is indicated in symptomatic patients. Either:

- *Transvenous balloon valvuloplasty*—potentially the treatment of choice in young patients with pliable non-calcified valves (indicated by echocardiography). The technique requires transeptal puncture and utilizes one (Inoue balloon) or two balloons. Inflation across the valve leads to an increase in valve orifice area and partial relief of stenosis (Fig. 103).
- *Mitral valve surgery*—open mitral valvotomy or mitral valve replacement continue to be needed in the majority of patients with symptomatic mitral stenosis.

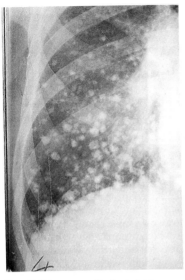

Fig. 100 Pulmonary ossification in long-standing mitral stenosis.

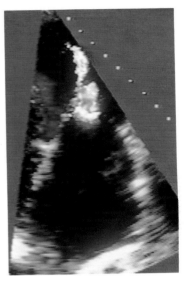

Fig. 101 Colour flow Doppler across the stenotic valve.

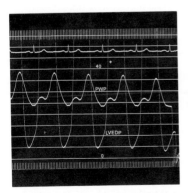

Fig. 102 Transvalvar gradient demonstrated between the LV and PWP at right and left heart catheterization.

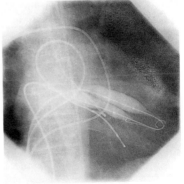

Fig. 103 Mitral valvuloplasty.

15 / Infective endocarditis

Definition | Infective endocarditis usually refers to bacterial infection of the heart valves. Infection with fungi (e.g. *Candida*), chlamydiae or rickettsiae also occurs although less frequently. Terms such as acute and subacute bacterial endocarditis (SBE) are now used less.

Incidence | Approximately 3000–4000 cases occur annually in the United Kingdom and the number may be increasing.

Risk factors | Any patient with damage to the endocardium is at increased risk of infective endocarditis. Those with valvular heart disease especially non-rheumatic (bicuspid aortic valves, mitral valve prolapse) and patients with congenital heart disease (e.g. ventricular septal defect, patent ductus arteriosus but not atrial septal defect) constitute the traditional high risk groups. New risk groups have become prominent and include intravenous drug abusers (right sided endocarditis more common) and those with prosthetic heart valves. Patients at risk should maintain good dental hygiene (Fig. 104) and receive antibiotic prophylaxis as recommended by national bodies.

Microbiology | A wide range of organisms can cause infective endocarditis. The commonest are viridans streptococci (Fig. 105): normal mouth flora whose surface glycoproteins enhance adherence to heart valves. Specific risk groups are prone to particular infections, e.g. the elderly to group D streptococci and intravenous drug addicts to *Staphylococcus* spp.

Pathology | Blood-borne organisms become lodged with platelets at the site of endocardial damage with the subsequent development of vegetations (Fig. 106). These can grow quite large particularly following infection with, for example, *Staphylococcus aureus* and fungi. Invasion into neighbouring structures can lead to valve incompetence (Fig. 107), conduction defects and abscess formation.

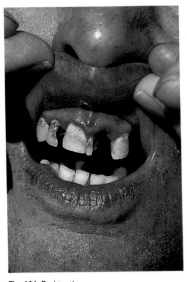

Fig. 104 Bad teeth.

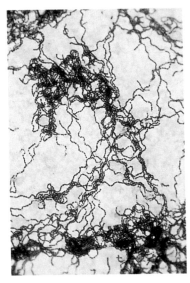

Fig. 105 *Streptococcus viridans*.

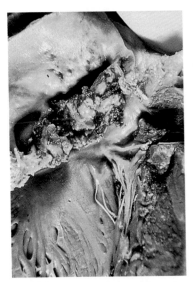

Fig. 106 Post-mortem pathology of the aortic valve showing extensive vegetations.

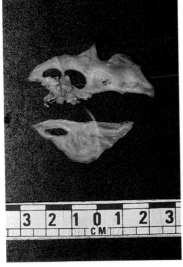

Fig. 107 Vegetations demonstrated clearly on aortic valve after removal at valve replacement.

Clinical recognition   Early diagnosis is the key to successful management. Relevant features in the history include an antecedent history of cardiac disease, recent dental or surgical procedures or a history of intravenous drug abuse. The diagnosis should be considered in any patient with unexplained fever, rashes, anaemia, murmurs or heart failure. A range of peripheral stigmata are described which may be relatively specific, e.g. Osler's nodes, Janeway lesions, or non-specific, e.g. clubbing (Fig. 108), petechiae (Fig. 109), leucocytoclastic vasculitis or splinter haemorrhages (Fig. 111).

Investigations   **Blood cultures.** If the diagnosis is a possibility then a series of blood cultures should be obtained and only then should intravenous antibiotics be commenced. The results of microbiology should not be awaited if there is reasonable clinical suspicion as it introduces unnecessary delay.

Electrocardiography. The ECG is important as conduction disturbances suggest extension of the infection into neighbouring myocardium (abscess).

Urine examination. Infective endocarditis may be complicated by renal involvement (usually glomerulonephritis) and urine microsopy is indicated in all patients.

Echocardiography. This allows early detection of vegetations (Fig. 110) or abscess formation and the development of other complications.

Management   Mortality from infective endocarditis remains high at approximately 20%. Choice of antibiotic and the duration of therapy should be decided in conjunction with a microbiologist. Intravenous therapy with antibiotics given in hospital remains standard practice. All patients should be reviewed by a cardiologist at an early stage, with valve surgery being indicated if there is haemodynamic deterioration, persistent infection, abscess formation, fungal or *Staph. aureus* infection, systemic emboli or large mobile vegetations.

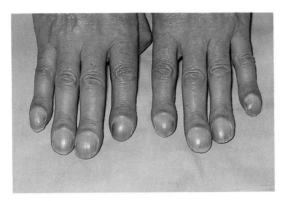

Fig. 108 Clubbing.

Fig. 109 Petechiae.

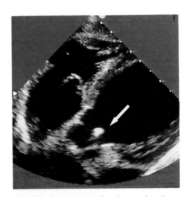

Fig. 110 Large vegetation the aortic valve.

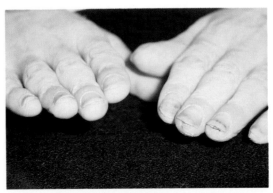

Fig. 111 Extensive splinter haemorrhages.

Acute pericarditis

Aetiology   Inflammation of the pericardium is most commonly due to infection with viruses, e.g. Coxsackie B, echo 8, mumps, influenza, Epstein–Barr. However, the range of causes is wide: bacterial, rheumatic diseases, neoplastic, uraemia and following myocardial infarction.

Clinical picture   The clinical syndrome is characterized by chest pain (retrosternal, radiating to the arms and shoulders and eased by sitting forward) and a friction rub.

Investigation   Serial repolarization changes on the ECG occur in 90% of cases (Fig. 112). ST elevation on the ECG is usually present in many leads and is concave upwards which serves to distinguish it from the ST changes of acute myocardial infarction. The chest X-ray is often normal, but echocardiography may reveal a small pericardial effusion.

Management   Management is symptomatic with anti-inflammatory analgesics and bed rest with the disease being self-limiting in the majority of patients.

Pericardial effusion

The development of an effusion in the pericardial space may occur with any inflammation of the pericardium.

Clinical picture   The effusion is often asymptomatic but large effusions with cardiac compression lead to cardiac tamponade with hypotension, pulsus paradoxus and an elevated jugular venous pressure.

Investigation   On the chest X-ray the cardiac silhouette does not usually widen until >250 ml fluid has accumulated. With a large effusion a globular appearance is characteristic (Fig. 113). Echocardiography provides the diagnosis (Fig. 114) and allows planning of optimal therapy.

Management   Pericardiocentesis is required to relieve haemodynamically significant effusions and obtain material for identification of cause. Chronic pericardial effusions, usually due to malignancy, may require open surgical drainage and the creation of a pericardial window and in some cases pericardiectomy.

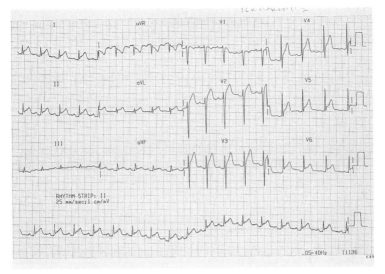

Fig. 112 Characteristic ECG of acute pericarditis.

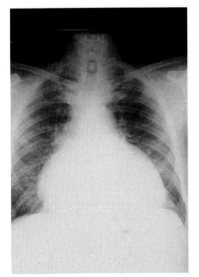

Fig. 113 Chest X-ray in patient with large pericardial effusion.

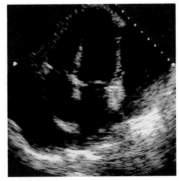

Fig. 114 2-D echocardiogram showing massive pericardial effusion (heart floating).

17 / Constrictive pericarditis

Definition   Constrictive pericarditis arises when a rigid inelastic pericardium adheres to the heart with impairment of diastolic filling. Diagnosis is often missed or delayed but is particularly important as surgical débridement of the pericardium results in cure.

Aetiology   Tuberculosis remains a common cause of constrictive pericarditis worldwide although it is an infrequent cause (<10%) in developed countries. Most cases now arise following previous cardiac surgery or mediastinal radiation although rheumatoid disease, previous viral infection or trauma can also result in pericardial constriction. Many cases remain idiopathic.

Clinical picture   Symptoms are usually those of heart failure with dyspnoea and oedema. Abdominal swelling with hepatomegaly and ascites more marked than peripheral oedema may lead to a mistaken diagnosis of liver disease. The key clinical signs are of a raised jugular venous pressure persisting despite diuretic therapy and an early 3rd heart sound (pericardial knock) on auscultation.

Investigation   The ECG typically shows reduced voltage (Fig. 115). Chest X-ray showing pericardial calcification on the lateral film is a useful clue but is not diagnostic of constriction (Figs 116 & 117). Findings on echocardiography are in general non-specific. The differential diagnosis from restrictive cardiomyopathy can be difficult since they produce similar haemodynamic derangements (Fig. 118). Differentiation depends on endomyocardial biopsy (perhaps showing amyloid infiltration) or on CT or magnetic resonance imaging scan (showing thickened pericardium).

Management   Patients with constrictive pericarditis benefit from complete surgical resection of the pericardium usually carried out under cardiopulmonary bypass. Operative mortality is, however, still as high as 5–10% in most centres.

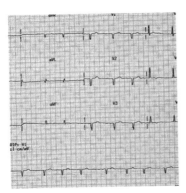

Fig. 115 Low voltage ECG.

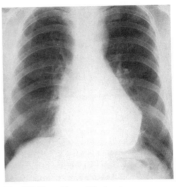

Fig. 116 Chest X-ray: PA showing pericardial calcification.

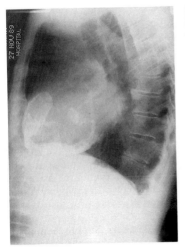

Fig. 117 Chest X-ray: lateral showing pericardial calcification.

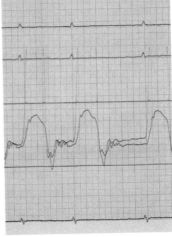

Fig. 118 Diastolic dip and plateau on simultaneous LV and RV pressure traces.

18 / Premature beats (extrasystoles)

Introduction The spectrum of abnormalities of cardiac rhythm ranges from benign, clinically insignificant disturbances of normal conduction to life-threatening arrhythmias. On a single ambulatory ECG recording more than 50% of normal individuals will have premature beats; at the dangerous end of the spectrum 50 Americans die every hour of malignant ventricular arrhythmia.

Definition Cardiac contractions initiated by ectopic foci occurring earlier than would otherwise be expected. The ventricles are the most common site of origin (Fig. 119) but contractions may arise from the atria, junctional zone or rarely the sinus node.

Clinical picture Frequency increase in the presence of structural heart disease. Premature beats are one of the most common causes of palpitation with heart beat being described as 'turning over' or 'skipping a beat'. They are usually noted at night or when the patient is otherwise at rest. Diagnosis may be suggested on the 12 lead ECG at the initial consultation (present on 1% of standard ECGs) but may need ambulatory recording (Fig. 120).

Significance Infrequent ventricular premature beats occurring in the absence of underlying heart disease are normal but become more frequent with increasing age. On the other hand, following myocardial infarction or in patients with structural heart disease, frequent (>10 per hour) complex premature ventricular beats are a bad prognostic sign. In these patients they serve principally as a marker of the severity of the underlying disorder. Suppression of ventricular permature beats alone does not improve prognosis and, indeed, in the Cardiac Arrhythma Suppression Trial, drug therapy increased mortality (Fig. 121), possibly by exacerbating the tendency to fatal arrhythmia (pro-arrhythmia).

Management The majority of patients need reassurance. Very symptomatic patients may benefit from drug therapy, beta-blockers being successful in many. In patients with symptomatic premature beats and underlying heart disease, the potentially serious side-effects of drug therapy such as pro-arrhythmia should be carefully weighed against the ill-defined benefits.

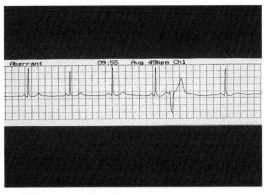

Fig. 119 Isolated ventricular ectopic.

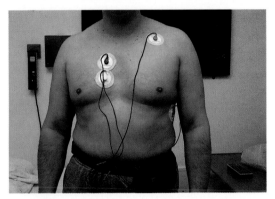

Fig. 120 Patient wearing Holter monitor.

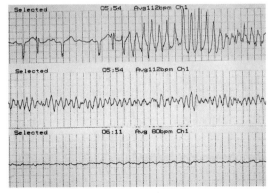

Fig. 121 Sinus rhythm leading to polymorphic VT, VF and asystole on ambulatory tape.

19 / **Paroxysmal supraventricular tachycardia (PSVT)**

This is a common arrhythmia which may present at any age including childhood and usually occurs in otherwise functionally normal hearts. The majority of patients with PSVT have *atrioventricular nodal re-entrant tachycardia* (AVNRT; Fig. 122) with a circus movement of depolarization in the atrioventricular node (junctional) region producing a regular narrow complex tachycardia. Re-entry may also occur via accessory atrioventricular pathways termed *atrioventricular re-entrant tachycardia* (AVRT) as in pre-excitation syndromes.

Presentation   A history of the sudden onset of rapid regular palpitations lasting for minutes to hours is characteristic. Vagotonic manoeuvres (e.g. Valsalva) may have been identified by the patient as being helpful in terminating symptoms. Dizziness, anxiety and breathlessness are relatively mild and only occasionally severe and incapacitating in patients with otherwise normal hearts. In patients with other cardiac disease, angina, heart failure or syncope may be precipitated.

Diagnosis   The 12 lead ECG in AVNRT is usually normal during sinus rhythm. Establishing the diagnosis requires an ECG recorded during an attack (12 lead ECG or obtained using ambulatory monitoring). In patients with infrequent attacks a patient-activated recording device may be necessary. Precise diagnosis requires electrophysiological study (EPS) (Figs 123 & 124), and this allows planning of optimal therapy in the symptomatic patient.

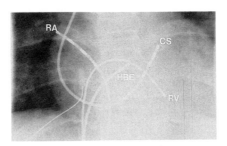

Fig. 122 PSVT — in this case AVRT with late retrograde atrial activation.

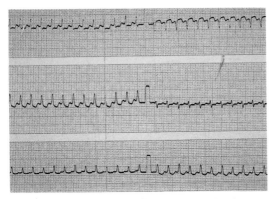

Fig. 123 EPS showing leads in place recording electrograms from right atrium (RA), right ventricle (RV), coronary sinus (CS) and His bundle (HBE).

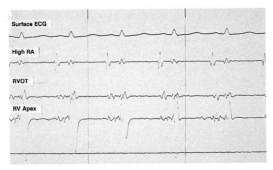

Fig. 124 Normal intracardiac electrogram, including RV outflow tract (RVOT).

Management **Termination.** Patients may present with tachycardia when the opportunity should be taken to record a 12 lead ECG. Arrhythmia termination may be attempted using vagotonic manoeuvres, but these are usually unsuccessful in those patients presenting to hospital. Drug termination should be attempted in the first instance using intravenous adenosine or verapamil. Supraventricular arrhythmias with aberrant conduction (wide QRS complex) are, for the purposes of immediate therapy, best regarded as rare and treatment should be as for ventricular tachycardia unless the diagnosis is certain.

Prophylaxis. Drug therapy is often tried for prophylaxis in patients with frequent episodes of arrhythmia but adequate suppression may prove difficult.

Cure. Patients remaining symptomatic on drug therapy can benefit from catheter modification of atrioventricular conduction. Alternatively some patients have benefited from the implantation of an antitachycardia pacemaker, although the use of these devices is now less common.

Pre-excitation syndromes

Pre-excitation is defined as early depolarization of ventricular myocardium via an alternative route bypassing the atrioventricular node. The Wolff–Parkinson–White (WPW) syndrome is the most common being characterized anatomically by an accessory connection(s) between atria and ventricles. Patients usually present with palpitations. The eponym refers to the ECG appearances (Fig. 125) in conjunction with symptoms and the incidence is unknown but the ECG abnormality is present in 0.03% of routine recordings. The 12 lead ECG in sinus rhythm shows a short PR interval and a delta wave (slurred onset of the QRS leading to wide complex). Symptomatic patients not responding to drug therapy require electrophysiological study. This identifies patients at risk of sudden death due to accelerated atrial fibrillation (Fig. 126). Radiofrequency catheter (Fig. 127) or surgical ablation of the accessory atrioventricular conduction pathway is indicated in the symptomatic patient.

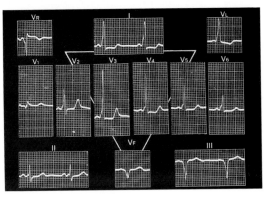

Fig. 125 Wolff–Parkinson–White ECG.

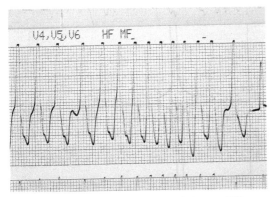

Fig. 126 Pre-excited atrial fibrillation — ventricular rate >300 bpm.

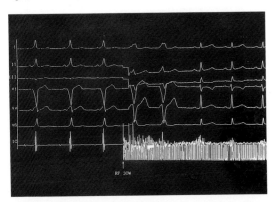

Fig. 127 Radiofrequency ablation in WPW—following ablation the delta wave disappears.

20 / **Atrial fibrillation (AF)**

Incidence   Atrial fibrillation is a very common arrhythmia affecting 2–5% of the population >60 years of age but may affect younger patients.

Definition   Atrial fibrillation is characterized by rapid disorganized atrial depolarization at rates exceeding 300/minute with an irregular ventricular response usually at rates exceeding 120/minute. The main consequences are decreased cardiac efficiency and an increased incidence of stroke.

Aetiology   Most patients with atrial fibrillation have underlying structural heart disease, usually coronary artery disease, rheumatic heart disease or chronic heart failure. Thyrotoxicosis (Fig. 128) should be considered as a cause in any patient even in the absence of other evidence of the disease (e.g. President George Bush). Occult thyroid disease may present in the elderly with atrial fibrillation. Infection, particularly pneumonia, pulmonary embolism, alcohol and bronchogenic carcinoma may all precipitate atrial fibrillation. Patients with no apparent cause, following a careful history and exclusion of structural heart disease and other causes, are said to have 'lone' atrial fibrillation.

Symptoms   These are dependent on a range of factors but especially on cardiac reserve and the dependence on atrial contraction for diastolic ventricular filling. A rapid ventricular response leads to decreased cardiac efficiency with a fall in cardiac output and symptoms of pulmonary congestion. Patients may present with an acute onset or, alternatively, with established arrhythmia with non-specific symptoms. Some patients have paroxysmal atrial fibrillation suggested initially by a clinical history of intermittent fast irregular palpitation and confirmed using ambulatory electrocardiography (Figs 129 & 130).

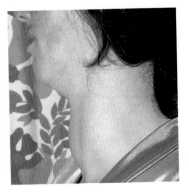

Fig. 128 Thyrotoxicosis.

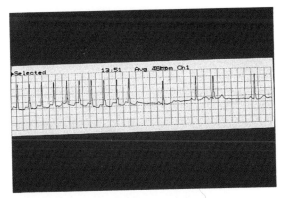

Fig. 129 Paroxysmal atrial fibrillation on ambulatory tape.

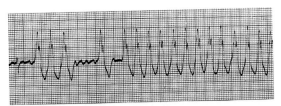

Fig. 130 Atrial fibrillation and ventricular tachycardia.

Investigations   All patients presenting with atrial fibrillation require a number of baseline investigations.

Electrocardiography. Although a presumptive diagnosis of atrial fibrillation can often be made clinically, the diagnosis is of such importance that an ECG should be obtained in all cases.

Thyroid function tests. These are essential in all patients even in the absence of other evidence of thyroid overactivity.

Echocardiography. This is an *essential* investigation in all patients with atrial fibrillation. It is important to exclude underlying valvular heart disease, assess left ventricular function and left atrial size and look for evidence of intracardiac thrombus (Fig. 131).

Complications   The principal complications are due to systemic embolism. Atrial fibrillation is a marker for patients at increased risk of stroke, usually embolic. The source of emboli is, however, often elsewhere in the vasculature such as the ascending aorta rather than the heart. Overall, the risk of stroke in atrial fibrillation is 5 times that of age-matched controls and, in patients with mitral stenosis, the risk increases to 25-fold. 20% of all strokes occur in patients with non-valvular atrial fibrillation.

Management   The principal aims are:

Control of ventricular rate. Digoxin remains the drug of choice and an absence of response should lead to a re-evaluation of the underlying cause or consideration of the possibility of inadequate dosing. Other atrioventricular nodal blocking drugs can be added.

Protection against systemic embolism. All patients with atrial fibrillation in association with valve disease should receive anticoagulation with warfarin. Other patients with non-valvular atrial fibrillation have often not been considered for anticoagulation but recent studies suggest a reduction of embolic events, in this group. Careful individualization of warfarin therapy reduces the risk of adverse effects from bleeding. Rare side-effects of warfarin include skin necrosis occurring in patients with coexistent procoagulant states such as protein S or C deficiency (Fig. 132).

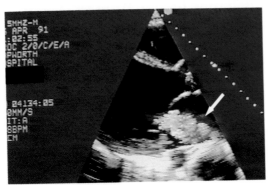

Fig. 131 Colour flow Doppler showing severe mitral regurgitation in a patient presenting with AF.

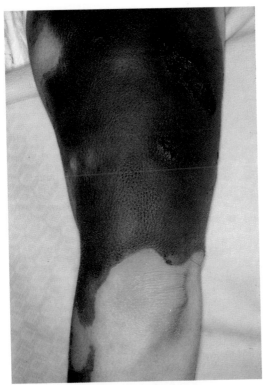

Fig. 132 Skin necrosis in patient with protein C deficiency given warfarin.

21 / Ventricular tachycardia (VT)

Definitions Five or more ventricular premature beats occurring consecutively define ventricular tachycardia. *Non-sustained ventricular tachycardia* (Fig. 133) terminates spontaneously in <30 seconds. *Sustained ventricular tachycardia* lasts >30 seconds or requires cardioversion to terminate the arrhythmia due to haemodynamic collapse.

Aetiology **Coronary artery disease.** Most patients with ventricular tachycardia have underlying coronary artery disease, and ventricular tachycardia may present early after myocardial infarction or later. The substrate is in the zone of the infarct scar being areas of slowed and dyshomogeneous conduction.

Cardiomyopathy. Dilated and hypertrophic cardiomyopathy predispose to the development of ventricular tachycardia which contributes to increased risk of sudden death in these conditions. Other causes include the long QT syndromes, drug induced arrhythmia and metabolic disturbances (e.g. magnesium deficiency) which all produce polymorphic VT (torsade de pointes) (Fig. 134) and right ventricular dysplasia. In some patients no underlying cause is identified.

Presentation Ventricular tachycardia may produce a range of symptoms. It may be asymptomatic or present with bouts of palpitations, dyspnoea or chest pain but more dramatic presentations with syncope are also common. The arrhythmia may be surprisingly well tolerated. In general, ventricular tachycardia is usually a bad prognostic marker and the first presentation of occult ventricular tachycardia may be sudden cardiac death.

Diagnosis Ventricular tachycardia is a 'broad complex tachycardia' and is by far the most common cause of this ECG pattern in older patients, especially if there is a preceding history of heart disease. Despite this, it continues to be confused with supraventricular tachycardia with aberrant conduction where management is radically different. The principal features in ventricular tachycardia distinguishing it from supraventricular arrhythmia are artrioventricular dissociation, very broad ORS complexes (>140 ms) and marked axis deviation (e.g. positive ORS complex in AVR).

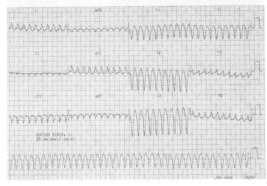

Fig. 133 Ventricular tachycardia.

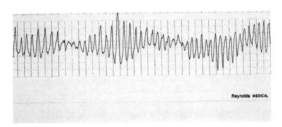

Fig. 134 Polymorphic ventricular tachycardia.

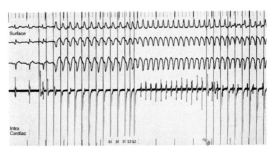

Fig. 135 Intracardiac electrogram recorded showing VT induction by pacing.

Investigations   Patients with ventricular tachycardia are at increased risk of sudden cardiac death (SCD) and require thorough investigation.

General. Estimation of structural and functional status of the heart with echocardiography, stress testing, coronary arteriography and measurement of ejection fraction is required in all patients.

Following myocardial infarction. Patients, following myocardial infarction, should be stratified in relation to their risk of serious ventricular arrhythmia. The assessment has often in the past relied on the use of ambulatory electrocardiography but the method lacks sensitivity. The use of more sophisticated screening tests such as heart rate variability, baroreflex sensitivity and the assessment of late potentials using signal averaged electrocardiography is being investigated.

Electrophysiological investigation. Patients presenting with sustained ventricular tachycardia or following resuscitation should be reviewed by a cardiologist with a view to more aggressive investigation possibly including programmed electrical stimulation (Fig. 135, p. 84).

Management   Management is complex and evolving, and best carried out by specialist electrophysiologists.

Pharmacological. Empiric drug therapy other than with amiodarone is generally not recommended. Drug therapy determined by serial electrophysiological testing is optimal. Amiodarone is highly effective but is complicated by side-effects, the most serious of which is pulmonary fibrosis.

Device therapy. Recent years have seen an exponential increase in the use of implanted devices to terminate ventricular tachycardia. Implantable cardioverter defibrillators (Figs 136 & 137) have an algorithm that recognizes the arrhythmia and then provides a defibrillating shock (Fig. 138). These devices can now use leads placed by transvenous insertion and their use is likely to increase. In most countries this will be constrained by the financial implications.

Curative therapy. Selected patients benefit from electrophysiologically guided surgery or catheter ablation to remove the arrhythmogenic substrate.

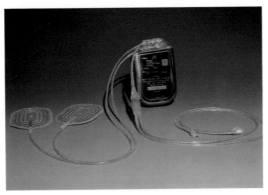

Fig. 136 Implantable cardioverter defibrillator.

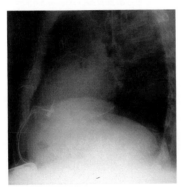

Fig. 137 Chest X-ray showing implantable defibrillator in abdominal position with patch electrodes.

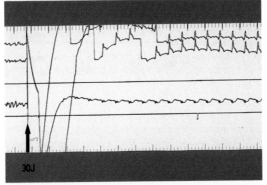

30J

Fig. 138 Implantable defibrillator recognizes VF (left) and gives defibrillatory shock converting to sinus rhythm.

22 / Cardiac syncope

1–3% of attendances in casualty departments and 3–6% of hospital admissions are for unexplained syncope.

Definition
Transient sudden loss of consciousness secondary to inadequate cerebral perfusion.

Aetiology
Simple fainting (vasovagal syncope) is the most common cause.

Arrhythmias. These should be considered in all patients. Bradycardia (Stokes–Adams attack) or tachycardia (e.g. ventricular tachycardia) may present with syncope.

Postural hypotension. This condition is often due to drug therapy in the elderly, for example overzealous use of diuretics and vasodilators, or occasionally due to autonomic failure (Parkinson's disease, Shy-Drager syndrome etc.).

Obstructive lesions. Patients with aortic stenosis, hypertrophic cardiomyopathy and pulmonary hypertension may present with syncope.

The main differential diagnosis is from epilepsy.

Investigation
The key to appropriate management of these patients is a careful history. Evidence of high degree atrioventricular block or other conduction anomaly may be present on the resting ECG (Fig. 139). Carotid sinus massage may reproduce symptoms and be associated with bradycardias. Ambulatory electrocardiography may reveal a specific cause such as ventricular tachycardia or paroxysmal atrioventricular block. In some patients further more sophisticated investigation such as electrophysiological testing may be necessary.

Tilt-induced syncope. Recently it has been recognized that some patients with otherwise unexplained syncope have symptoms reproducible by head-up tilt, most easily achieved using a table designed for the purpose (Fig. 140).

Management
Patients with syncope due to bradycardia will benefit from the insertion of a pacemaker. In other patients even after extensive investigations no specific cause is identified. The outlook for survival in these patients is excellent although morbidity may remain high (Fig. 141).

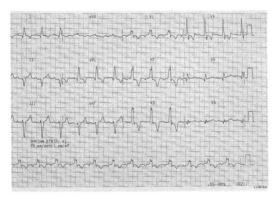

Fig. 139 Trifascicular block in patient with syncope needing pacemaker.

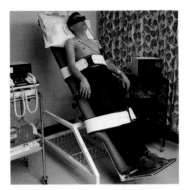

Fig. 140 Tilt table.

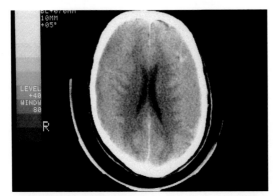

Fig. 141 Subdural haematoma seen on CT scan as isodense shadow in patient with head injury due to Stokes–Adams attack.

23 / Pacemakers

Pacemakers are highly cost effective. In appropriate patients, pacing cures symptoms and improves prognosis. More than 1.5 million pacemakers have now been implanted worldwide; however, the use of pacemakers differs significantly between countries. In the mid 1980s use in sinoatrial disease in the US was 8 times that of the UK. Despite the US implantation rate declining by 25% in the late 1980s rates are still considerably in excess of those in the UK. Implantation rate in the UK averaged 148/million (1986) and in the US and other European countries it is around 350/million. These countries also use more appropriate pacemaker types.

Indications   The main considerations are the improvement of symptoms and the prognosis.

Atrioventricular block. All patients with symptomatic congenital complete heart block should be paced. Patients with acquired complete heart block (and probably those with 2nd degree AV block) should all receive a pacemaker, whether symptomatic or not, in order to improve prognosis (Fig. 142).

Sinoatrial disease (sick sinus syndrome). These patients should receive a pacemaker if they have symptomatic bradycardia.

Presentation   **Asymptomatic.** Any patient found to have complete heart block should be referred for pacemaker implantation.

Symptomatic bradycardia. Patients with a slow pulse and dizzy spells, fatigue, dyspnoea, or congestive heart failure usually benefit from pacemaker implantation.

Stokes–Adams attacks. The presentation of a patient with syncope and a history compatible with Stokes–Adams attack should lead to a full investigation. Evidence of complete heart block is an absolute indication for the early implantation of a permanent pacemaker.

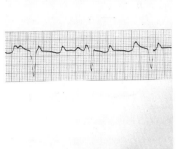

Fig. 142 Complete heart block.

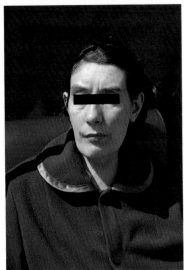

Fig. 143 Dystrophia myotonica.

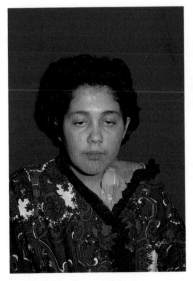

Fig. 144 Kearns–Sayre syndrome.

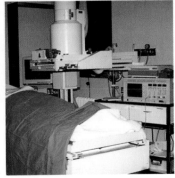

Fig. 145 Pacing room.

Aetiology   The majority of patients that need pacemakers have idiopathic degeneration of part of the cardiac conducting system. Coronary artery disease may be the underlying problem. In addition some patients with skeletal and heart muscle disease (e.g. dystrophia myotonica; Fig. 143, p. 90) may develop heart block. Kearns–Sayre syndrome (Fig. 144, p. 90) is the rare combination of progressive external ophthalmoplegia, retinal pigmentary degeneration and progressive impairment of cardiac conduction. Other causes of heart block that should be considered particularly in younger patients include infiltrative disease such as sarcoidosis, rheumatoid or amyloid and infections such as Lyme disease.

Procedure   Implantation of a pacemaker is a relatively straightforward procedure under local anaesthetic (Fig. 145, p. 90). The pacemaker lead is advanced to the apex of the right ventricle, usually from the cephalic or subclavian vein, and the pacemaker generator is then placed subcutaneously on the anterior chest wall. The procedure is usually undertaken as an inpatient with the patient remaining in hospital for approximately 48 hours.

Pacemaker types

An international code has been established to describe available pacemaker types (Fig. 146). The most common types of pacemaker in use in the UK are ventricular demand units (VVI; Fig. 147) which are relatively inexpensive, but reliable and able to prevent major symptoms of syncope and improve prognosis. Because VVI pacemakers do not provide coordinated atrial and ventricular contraction or increase pacing rate on exercise they are not optimal in most patients. Rate responsive pacemakers (VVIR) have a sensor that increases the rate of discharge with physical activity. Dual chamber pacemakers (DDD; Fig. 148) sense and pace both atrium and ventricle and provide atrioventricular coordination, being able to 'track' the normal sinus rate on exercise (Fig. 149). Two pacing wires are required but they provide a more physiological replacement of the normal conducting system.

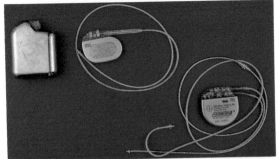

Fig. 146 Pacemaker types (old fashioned generator, WI and DDD pacemaker with leads attached).

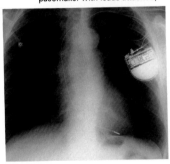

Fig. 147 VVI pacemaker (single lead).

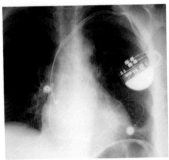

Fig. 148 DDD pacemaker (atrial and ventricular leads).

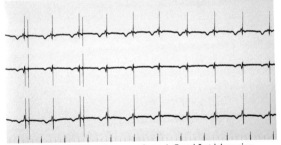

Fig. 149 ECG of DDD pacing: complexes 1–7 and 9 atrial sensing with trigged ventricular pacing; complexes 8–10 atrial and ventricular pacing.

Complications of pacemaker implantation

If a patient presents with unexplained symptoms following pacemaker insertion then the pacing centre responsible for that patient should be contacted immediately.

Early complications

Lead displacement. The patient may present with a recurrence of the initial symptoms if the primary problem is loss of capture; if the problem is a failure to sense intrinsic cardiac activity then palpitations are more usual.

Early or late complications

Myoinhibition. Some patients complain of dizziness and, occasionally, syncope on arm movement due to myoinhibition where activity of the pectoral muscles is detected by the pacemaker leading to an inappropriate reduction of pacemaker discharge.

Infection. An infection develops in 1–2% of patients and presents with pain over the pacemaker site if the pacemaker pocket is involved. If the system itself is infected the entire unit must be removed (Fig. 150). Infection usually presents in the first few weeks following implantation but occasionally much later.

Thrombosis. Oedema of the arm on the side of pacemaker insertion may occur (<1% of patients) and if severe may be improved by warfarinization.

Pacemaker syndrome. This is a major disadvantage of VVI pacing. The condition is characterized by dizziness and heavy palpitations due to loss of properly timed atrial systole. Cure usually follows upgrade to a dual chamber system.

Late complications

Lead fracture or battery failure. The patient usually presents with recurrence of the initial symptoms and requires change of the generator or the entire system.

Erosion. The generator or wire may erode through the overlying skin (Fig. 151) inevitably leading to infection. Early surgery is needed to limit the spread of infection.

Superior vena cava syndrome. Rarely, patients develop stenosis of the superior vena cava with symptoms including swelling of the upper body and headache (Fig. 152).

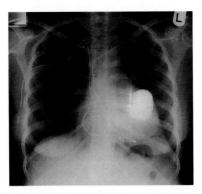

Fig. 150 Multiple pacemaker leads following many complications and procedures.

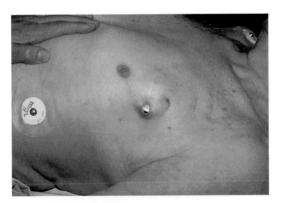

Fig. 151 Erosion of pacemaker generator through the skin.

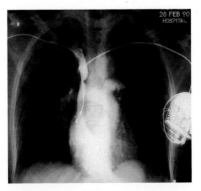

Fig. 152 SVC stenosis due to pacemaker lead.

24 / Atrial septal defect (ASD)

The most common (30%) congenital heart abnormality detected in adult patients although it constitutes 6% of congenital heart disease in children.

Classification **Ostium secundum:** common type occurring in 70% of cases. Located in the fossa ovalis, it occurs more commonly in females (ratio 3:1) and 20–30% have associated mitral valve prolapse.

Sinus venosus: (15% of total) occurring in upper portion of the interatrial septum and often accompanied by partial anomalous pulmonary venous drainage.

Ostium primum: sited in the lower septum. This type most commonly presents in childhood (often in Down syndrome) and is usually associated with other abnormalities (Fig. 153).

Presentation Adults present with fatigue, dyspnoea, palpitations and chest pain. The presentation may be associated with the onset of atrial fibrillation.

Signs The most characteristic finding is of wide fixed splitting of the second heart sound. Pulmonary and tricuspid flow murmurs are usual.

Investigations **Chest X-ray:** in uncomplicated cases shows a small aortic knuckle and pulmonary plethora (Fig. 154). Later right sided chambers may become dilated indicating impending right heart failure.

Electrocardiography: ostium secundum ASD often has right bundle branch block, usually incomplete (rSr′ complex with QRS <0.10 s), and right axis deviation.

Echocardiography: investigation of choice. The defect is demonstrated along with right ventricular volume overload and paradoxical septal motion. Doppler echo will localize the defect (Fig. 155).

Right heart catheterization: demonstrates 'step up' in oxygen saturation between the venae cavae and the right ventricle.

Management Operative closure is usually recommended if pulmonary to systemic blood flow ratio >1.5:1. Operation will reverse haemodynamic abnormalities (Fig. 156) and prevent complications of right heart failure, paradoxical embolism and pulmonary vascular disease.

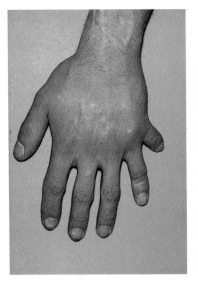

Fig. 153 Multiple digits may occur in patients with ASD.

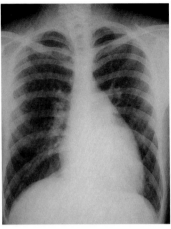

Fig. 154 Preoperative chest X-ray showing plethora due to increased pulmonary blood flow.

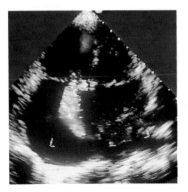

Fig. 155 Colour flow Doppler with flow across large defect.

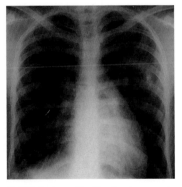

Fig. 156 Postoperative film showing normal lung fields.

25 / Ventricular septal defect (VSD)

Most common congenital heart defect (30%) although the majority are detected before adulthood due to prominent physical signs. In addition to occurring as a congenital abnormality the defect may complicate acute myocardial infarction.

Anatomy The defect may occur anywhere along the ventricular septum but most commonly in the membranous septum (infracristal) occurring in 70%. It may be part of Down's syndrome often in association with an ASD.

Presentation The presentation of VSD in adulthood is rare but usually follows the finding of a murmur or the development of complications.

Signs The classic murmur is harsh and pansystolic and sited at the lower left sternal edge. An accompanying thrill is usual. 5–10% have aortic regurgitation due to prolapse of a valve leaflet into the defect.

Investigation Diagnosis is by echocardiography. Identification of small defects (Maladie de Roger) is facilitated by the use of colour flow Doppler studies. Chest X-ray appearances are non-specific but demonstrate pulmonary plethora due to increased pulmonary blood flow.

Management Patients with small defects are managed expectantly with a greater than 30% chance of spontaneous closure in young patients. Large defects with a ratio of pulmonary to systemic flow >2:1 and right ventricular overload need surgical closure. Patients are at risk of endocarditis and should receive appropriate advice about antibiotics.

Fallot's tetralogy

Most common form of cyanotic congenital heart disease (Fig. 157). Consists of pulmonary stenosis or atresia, ventricular septal defect, dextroposition of the aorta overriding the septal defect and right ventricular hypertrophy. Survival into adulthood is now common, although patients remain at considerable risk of a range of complications.

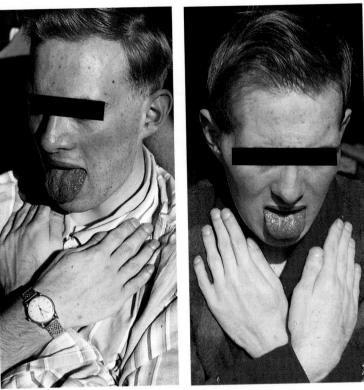

Fig. 157 Patient with Fallot's tetralogy benefits from complete repair with disappearance of cyanosis.

26 / Pulmonary stenosis (PS)

This condition constitutes 10–12% of congenital heart disease. Acquired PS is unusual but may occur in rheumatic heart disease, following trauma and rarely due to the carcinoid syndrome (tricuspid stenosis with regurgitation is more common). Pulmonary stenosis may be part of Noonan syndrome (Fig. 158).

Presentation   Usually asymptomatic but may present with dyspnoea, easy fatiguability and occasionally chest pain and syncope on exertion.

Signs   The key physical finding is of a systolic murmur at the upper left sternal edge. An ejection click is often present and the second heart sound is soft and delayed. There is usually a thrill in the same area.

Investigation   ***Chest X-ray:*** pulmonary artery dilated and pulmonary vascular markings may be diminished with severe pulmonary stenosis (Fig. 159). The right ventricle may be enlarged and occasionally markedly so.

Electrocardiography: demonstrates right axis deviation, bundle branch block and ventricular hypertrophy.

Echocardiography: provides the diagnosis with Doppler allowing estimation of the transvalvar gradient and hence quantification of severity.

Right heart catheterization: gradient is observed on withdrawal across the stenosis. Right ventricular angiography shows doming of the valve.

Management   Asymptomatic patients with mild to moderate stenosis do not need treatment and as the valve lesion is non-progressive are unlikely to do so. Patients with moderate or severe stenosis (gradient >60 mmHg) and symptoms, or with evidence of right ventricular dysfunction, usually need treatment. This is now most efficiently carried out using transvenous balloon valvuloplasty (Fig. 160).

Peripheral pulmonic stenosis

Some patients have supravalvular pulmonary stenosis (Fig. 161) and this occasionally may consist of multiple narrowings of the primary and more peripheral branches and is often a part of the rubella syndrome.

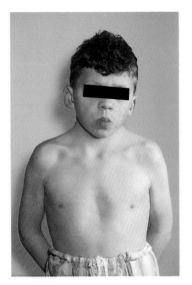

Fig. 158 Noonan syndrome.

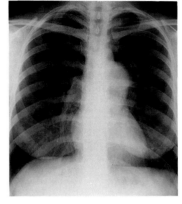

Fig. 159 Typical chest X-ray appearance.

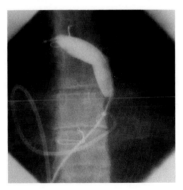

Fig. 160 Pulmonary balloon valvuloplasty.

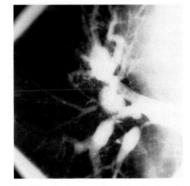

Fig. 161 Angiogram of peripheral pulmonic stenoses.

27 / Coarctation

Coarctation of the aorta is due to a localized shelf-like thickening of the aortic wall usually opposite the ligamentum arteriosum. Males are affected twice as commonly as females.

Associations There is high degree of association with gonadal dysgenesis (Turner syndrome; Fig. 162) and also with bicuspid aortic valve.

Presentation Most adults with coarctation are asymptomatic but may have headache, claudication or fatigue. Coarctation is usually detected on routine examination with hypertension and diminished femoral pulses. Signs of a bicuspid aortic valve may be present (30%). A murmur is often present over the back due to collateral flow.

Investigations **Electrocardiography.** Evidence of left ventricular hypertrophy is often present.

Chest X-ray. Left ventricular enlargement is possible but notching on the lower posterior border of the 3rd to 8th ribs is common (Fig. 163). Pre- and post-stenotic dilatation of the aorta around the site of the narrowing may be seen.

Aortography. This identifies site of obstruction (Fig. 164), demonstrates extent of collateral filling and also allows measurement of the pressure gradient across the stenosis (Fig. 165).

Natural history Mean life expectancy without treatment is 35 years. Death is most commonly the result of the complications of hypertension especially cerebrovascular disease (sub-arachnoid haemorrhage is common due to the increased incidence of berry aneurysms), left ventricular failure or aortic dissection. Improvement in prognosis is achieved with surgery although hypertension usually remains postoperatively if the patient is >5 years old. In one study 70% of patients were hypertensive 30 years following surgery.

Treatment Surgery remains the treatment of choice; long-term follow-up is essential. Recurrence of coarctation is possible and complications arising from previous hypertension and associated valve lesions are common.

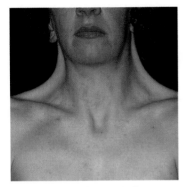

Fig. 162 Webbing of the neck in Turner syndrome.

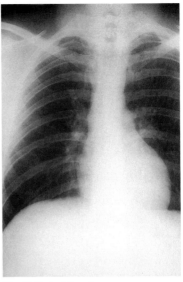

Fig. 163 Typical chest X-ray.

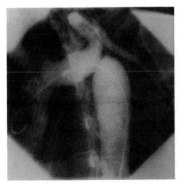

Fig. 164 Aortogram.

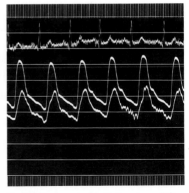

Fig. 165 Pressure gradient between arm (left brachial artery) and leg (left femoral artery).

28 / Patent ductus arteriosus (PDA); sinus of Valsalva fistula

Patent ductus arteriosus (PDA)

Definition Persistent arterial channel connecting the aortic isthmus to the left pulmonary artery, now seen rarely in adults.

Presentation The anomaly is usually asymptomatic but there is a risk of developing heart failure, shunt reversal with development of Eisenmenger syndrome and bacterial endarteritis each of which may bring the condition to light.

Diagnosis Continuous (machinery) murmur is of maximal intensity in the 2nd left intercostal interspace and may be the first clue to the problem.

Chest X-ray: may show cardiac enlargement and pulmonary plethora. Calcification of the ductus may lead to a characteristic appearance in older patients.

Management Ligation of the duct or, more usually in adults, resection are truly curative if carried out prior to a rise in pulmonary artery pressure. Treatment is indicated in all patients to reduce the risk of complications.

Sinus of Valsalva fistula

This condition is rare but is the second most common cause of a continuous murmur in adult patients. Sinus aneurysms are either congenital or can occur secondary to infective endocarditis. Rupture usually occurs into the right ventricle and is associated with an acute attack of chest pain and possibly acute heart failure. The murmur is heard best in the second right intercostal space in most cases. Colour flow Doppler is diagnostic and the lesion can also be demonstrated by aortography (Fig. 166). Surgical closure reduces the risk of ventricular dysfunction, infective endocarditis, septic pulmonary embolism and shunt reversal.

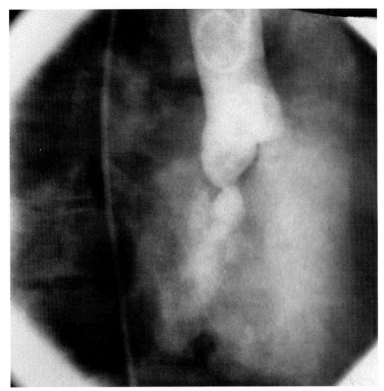

Fig. 166 Aortogram of sinus of Valsalva fistula showing flow between the right coronary sinus and the right ventricle.

29 / **Eisenmenger syndrome**

Definition   Eisenmenger complex refers to ventricular septal defect with pulmonary hypertension and right to left shunting of blood through the defect leading to systemic desaturation. Eisenmenger syndrome occurs following reversal of any left to right shunt (usually VSD, PDA, atrioventricular septal defect and unusually ostium secundum ASD) following the development of pulmonary hypertension. Pulmonary hypertension develops due to thickening of the walls of the pulmonary arterial bed the precise mechanisms of which are not established.

Clinical picture   Associated with symptoms of dyspnoea, easy fatiguability and haemoptysis. Cyanosis and clubbing are present. The unusual appearance of differential cyanosis with blue clubbed toes and pink lips and fingers occurs following shunt reversal through a PDA (Fig. 167). Chest X-ray appearances may be bizarre with a very prominent pulmonary trunk and pulmonary arteries with peripheral oligaemia ('tree in winter') and evidence of right ventricular enlargement is often present (Fig. 168).

Management   Individuals with cyanotic congenital heart disease including Eisenmenger syndrome commonly survive into adulthood. These patients have a number of special problems needing careful management. These include polycythaemia (need regular venesection), gout (prophylactic allopurinol often indicated), contraceptive advice (pregnancy usually poorly tolerated) and endocarditis. They often benefit from follow-up in a specialist clinic. Overall life expectancy is shortened. Selected patients may be candidates for heart–lung transplantation.

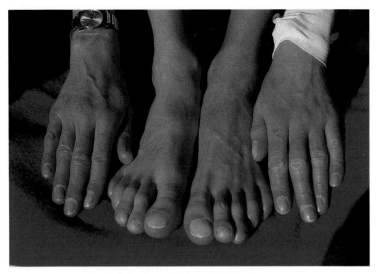

Fig. 167 Differential cyanosis and clubbing in patient with Eisenmenger PDA.

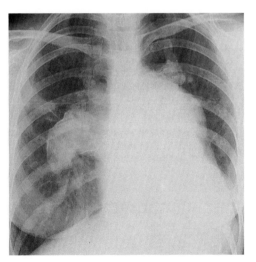

Fig. 168 Chest X-ray of Eisenmenger syndrome (ASD).

Thoracic aortic aneurysms

Aneurysms of the thoracic aorta are relatively uncommon and due to a number of causes.

Aetiology

Arteriosclerosis: the most common cause and may develop in any part of the thoracic aorta. The entire aorta may be ectatic and usually there is widespread arteriosclerosis elsewhere. The aneurysm itself is usually fusiform.

Cystic medial necrosis: may result in annuloaortic ectasia and is a common component of the Marfan syndrome (Fig. 169) and Ehlers–Danlos syndrome. Aortic dissection, rupture or regurgitation may develop. Annuloaortic ectasia is present in 5–10% of patients requiring aortic valve replacement.

Syphilis: luetic aneurysms develop in 5–10% of patients with syphilitic aortitis. Patients develop a destructive aortitis which involves both the ascending aorta and the arch. Aortic regurgitation commonly develops due to involvement of the aortic valve cusps, and angina may occur due to coronary ostial stenosis. Aneurysms may become huge and erode the sternum and ribs (Figs 170 & 171). On the chest X-ray, calcification is usually present in the aneurysm wall.

Management

Most patients are asymptomatic and come to light following a routine chest X-ray. Prophylactic surgical replacement is often needed in patients with large aneurysms but may carry significant risks (Fig. 172).

Aortitis

Inflammation of the wall of the aorta is termed aortitis and may occur for a host of reasons. Syphilis is a well-recognized cause but is now uncommon. Other causes include ankylosing spondylitis, Reiter's syndrome, ulcerative colitis and Takayasu's arteritis.

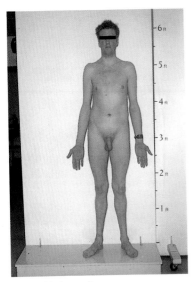

Fig. 169 Marfan syndrome.

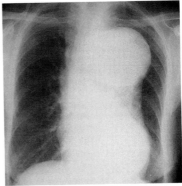

Fig. 170 Huge luetic aneurysm—chest X-ray.

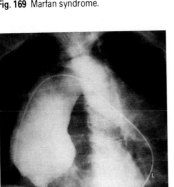

Fig. 171 An aortogram of the same aneurysm in Fig. 170.

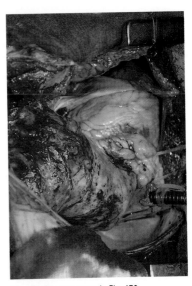

Fig. 172 The aneurysm in Fig. 170—intraoperative.

31 / **Aortic dissection**

Description   Aortic intimal tear followed by tracking of blood into the aortic media (Fig. 173). The usual site is the ascending aorta (type A) but other sites of origin are possible. Predisposing causes include hypertension (70–90% of patients have history of hypertension), Marfan syndrome (Fig. 174), Ehlers–Danlos syndrome, bicuspid aortic valve and chest trauma. Males are affected more commonly than females (3:1) but dissection is described, for example, in pregnancy.

Presentation   Sudden onset of severe precordial or interscapular pain is characteristic. Blood pressure is often increased (in 50–70%) despite a shock-like state. An early diastolic murmur may be present. Crucial differential diagnosis is from acute myocardial infarction as thrombolytic treatment in dissection proves catastrophic.

Investigation   ***Chest X-ray.*** Abnormal in 80% with mediastinal widening (Fig. 175) and left pleural effusion being the most common. However, the chest X-ray may be normal.
Electrocardiography. This usually shows left ventricular hypertrophy resulting from hypertension but there are no specific changes. It helps to exclude other causes of chest pain particularly myocardial infarction which may coexist with dissection (due to obstruction of the coronary ostia) although this is rare.
Definitive diagnosis. Thoracic aortography (Fig. 176) remains the investigation of choice in many centres. Transoesophageal echocardiography may provide more information but is of limited availability. Thoracic CT scanning and MRI can also be used.

Management   Medical treatment is with analgesia and reduction of heart rate and blood pressure with beta-blockers and sodium nitroprusside. Immediate surgery is required in all patients with acute dissection of the ascending aorta. The ascending aorta is replaced with a prosthetic graft and the false channel obliterated. Operative mortality remains, however, around 50%. Surgery for distal (type B) dissection is usually reserved for patients developing complications or those with the Marfan syndrome.

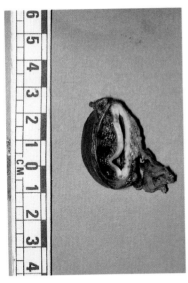

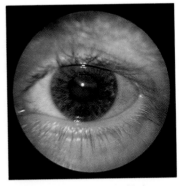

Fig. 173 Dissecting aneurysm (post-mortem) with tracking of blood in the media and partial obliteration of the lumen.

Fig. 174 Lens dislocation in the Marfan syndrome.

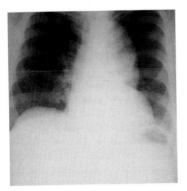

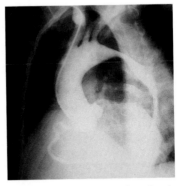

Fig. 175 Chest X-ray showing widened mediastinum.

Fig. 176 Aortography showing dissection of the arch.

32 / Pulmonary embolism

Definition Complication of venous thrombosis usually arising in the deep veins of the legs. Some patients postoperatively are at particular risk (e.g. increased age, immobility, malignancy).

Symptoms Clinical diagnosis lacks both sensitivity and specificity. Symptoms may include dyspnoea on exertion and at rest, pleuritic or central chest pain, haemoptysis and syncope.

Signs On examination the patient may have tachypnoea, be using accessory muscles, have a friction rub, a left parasternal heave, raised venous pressure and tachycardia or no signs whatsoever.

Investigations **Chest X-ray:** often normal and findings when present are non-specific, e.g. basal atelectasis. Chest X-ray is most helpful in demonstrating another cause for the patient's clinical presentation such as pneumothorax, pneumonia, pulmonary oedema etc.

Electrocardiography: often normal (>30%). Changes such as $S_1Q_3T_3$ and RBBB are non-specific. The ECG may serve to exclude other possible causes of symptoms, e.g. myocardial infarction.

Lung scanning: perfusion or ventilation–perfusion scanning (Fig. 177) often useful as initial diagnostic test. Mismatching of ventilation and perfusion with pulmonary embolism (Fig. 178) is a useful pointer but is not specific.

Pulmonary angiography: reference standard for the diagnosis of pulmonary embolism. Emboli are demonstrated as constant filling defects with sharp cut off (Fig. 179).

Management The majority of patients require anticoagulation, initially with heparin and subsequently with warfarin. Patients with massive pulmonary embolism may be candidates for more aggressive therapy with thrombolytic agents or pulmonary embolectomy. Fragmentation of an embolus with the tip of a pulmonary catheter can speed dissolution. Prevention of the passage of further clot from the deep venous system may be aided by the insertion of a caval filter (Fig. 180).

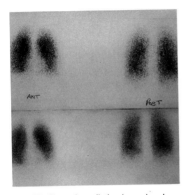

Fig. 177 Normal ventilation (upper) and perfusion (lower) scans.

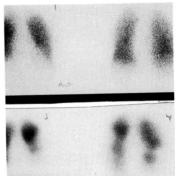

Fig. 178 Mismatch of ventilation and perfusion with multiple pulmonary emboli.

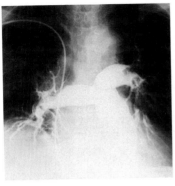

Fig. 179 Pulmonary angiogram showing filling defect and sharp cut off typical of pulmonary embolism.

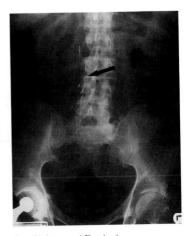

Fig. 180 Intracaval filter in situ.

33 / Primary pulmonary hypertension

Pulmonary hypertension is defined by the presence of a high pulmonary artery pressure reflecting increased pulmonary vascular resistance. In many patients no specific cause is identified and the condition is termed primary pulmonary hypertension.

Clinical picture The condition affects females more than males (5:1). Patients are usually aged 15–40, and present with fatigue and exertional syncope, but chest pain or dyspnoea may dominate. Patients may have evidence of a connective tissue disease, with Raynaud's phenomenon, and may have a malar flush. Patients usually have peripheral, but not central, cyanosis when at rest, and may have an 'a' wave visible in the venous pulse, a right ventricular heave and (on auscultation) a loud pulmonary component of the second heart sound.

Investigations **Chest X-ray:** may show cardiomegaly with enlargement of the right sided chambers (Fig. 181), the pulmonary artery is enlarged with peripheral oligaemia ('pruning'), the aortic knuckle may appear relatively small.

Echocardiography: demonstrates a dilated right ventricle (Fig. 182) and paradoxical septal motion.

Right heart catheterization: confirms diagnosis of pulmonary hypertension with a raised pulmonary artery pressure. Mixed venous oxygen saturation and cardiac output correlate with prognosis.

Pulmonary angiography: usually required to exclude large vessel proximal thromboembolism that may be helped with thrombendarterectomy.

Lung biopsy: definitive diagnostic test (Fig. 183), although similar changes can occur in Eisenmenger complex, with muscle hypertrophy, constriction and hypoplasia of peripheral pulmonary arteries (plexiform lesions).

Natural history Although spontaneous remission has been reported the usual tendency is to a progressive downhill course with 10-year survival being <25%.

Management Most patients should receive anticoagulants, and a trial of vasodilator therapy may be attempted with caution. Heart–lung transplantation may be considered.

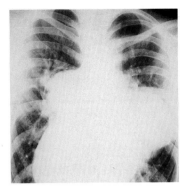

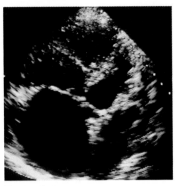

Fig. 181 Chest X-ray; primary pulmonary hypertension with massive proximal pulmonary arteries.

Fig. 182 Right ventricular enlargement on 2-D echocardiogram (large dark space lower left).

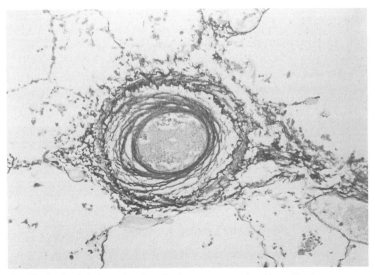

Fig. 183 Intraluminal obstruction of small pulmonary artery — lung biopsy histology.

34 / Cardiac tumours

75% of cardiac tumours are benign. The most common by far is myxoma but lipomas, fibroelastoma and rhabdomyoma also can occur.

Atrial myxoma

Myxomas are thought to arise from primitive mesenchymal cells. 90% arise in the atria, four times more commonly on the left than the right. They are pedunculated and attached to the interatrial septum at the fossa ovalis.

Clinical picture   Patients may present at any age. In some the condition is familial. Patients may be asymptomatic, present with symptoms of mitral stenosis, with symptoms of systemic embolism or with lethargy, fevers etc. Findings on examination can be similar to those in mitral stenosis.

Investigation   Routine laboratory tests may be abnormal with normochromic normocytic anaemia, leucocytosis, raised ESR and immunoglobulins. Chest X-ray appearances may resemble those of mitral stenosis though the left atrial appendage is not so prominent. The tumour may be calcified. Echocardiography is the investigation of choice (Fig. 184). Angiography is no longer required but may produce dramatic images (Fig. 185).

Management   Complete surgical resection (Fig. 186) is the treatment of choice.

Malignant cardiac tumours

The most common are directly invasive from lung primaries or secondary deposits from elsewhere. Sarcomas are the most common primary cardiac tumours and present with heart failure, arrhythmias and effusions. The prognosis in these patients is extremely poor.

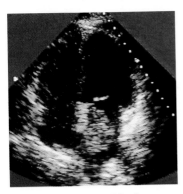

Fig. 184 Atrial myxoma on 2-D echo.

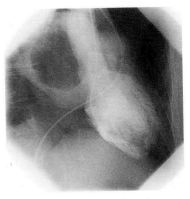

Fig. 185 Atrial myxoma on angiography shown as large filling defect after mitral reflux from LV angiogram.

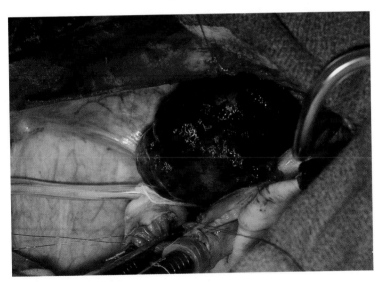

Fig. 186 Removal of atrial myxoma.

35 / Heart in hypertension

Left ventricular hypertrophy in hypertension is both an adaptive response to increased work and an adverse prognostic indicator.

Incidence ECG evidence of left ventricular hypertrophy is found in 15% of unselected patients with mild hypertension, 50% of patients with mild to moderate hypertension and 90% of patients admitted to hospital with hypertension. Left ventricular hypertrophy is 10 times more prevalent in patients with blood pressure >160/95 than in the normotensive population. Hypertrophy is usually concentric with an increase in wall thickness and no increase in chamber size.

Detection **Electrocardiography:** standard method of detection (Fig. 187) but lacks sensitivity. Standard criteria sum voltages from R wave in V_1 or V_2 and S wave in V_5 or V_6 which should not exceed 35 mm. Repolarization changes commonly accompany these changes.

Echocardiography: increased wall thickness or muscle mass on echo is now taken as the standard index of left ventricular hypertrophy (Fig. 188) for epidemiological or clinical studies.

Consequences The presence of left ventricular hypertrophy increases the risk of fatal events in both male and female patients with hypertension. Presence of left ventricular hypertrophy in men aged 35–64 increases risk more than 7-fold. Eventually hypertrophy leads to impairment of relaxation and heart failure. Although not proven, a reduction in left ventricular mass with antihypertensive therapy (Fig. 189) may have a beneficial effect on prognosis.

Heart failure

Heart failure occurs in hypertension as a result of increased workload, direct myocyte necrosis and decreases in coronary vascular reserve. The incidence of heart failure arising as a consequence of hypertension has decreased dramatically probably as a function of improved detection and treatment of hypertension. When hypertension is due to phaeochromocytoma (Fig. 190) then sudden surges of blood pressure may lead to acute heart failure.

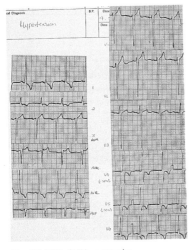

Fig. 187 ECG of LV hypertrophy.

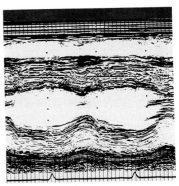

Fig. 188 M-mode echocardiogram of concentric LV hypertrophy with thickened septum and posterior wall.

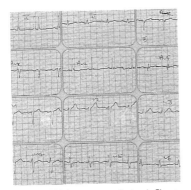

Fig. 189 ECG from same patient as in Figure 187 on treatment 12 years later showing evidence of regression of LV hypertrophy.

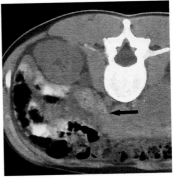

Fig. 190 Phaeochromocytoma: right renal hilum.

Index